Praise For *I've Been Thinking*
By Frank J. Weinstock, M.D., F.A.C.S.

"Dr. Frank Weinstock's book condenses a lifetime of experience as a physician into an easy-to-read text that can help consumers navigate the complexities of health care in the United States. It stresses the importance of individuals taking responsibility for their own health and health care decisions, and it provides guidance on how best to do so. The information about eye care is especially complete and compelling."

—C. William Keck, M.D., M.P.H., *Professor Emeritus Northeast Ohio Medical University*

"So much of our day-to-day conversation involves matters related to health and America's confusing and costly health care system; and, few things are more precious to us than our good health and the good health of those we love. Fortunately, because of medical research and recent advances in medical technologies, we now have tools which enable us to prevent illness and, if we get sick, the ability to regain good health. But the "health care system" is so complex and confusing that many people feel overwhelmed and unable to cope with it. That's why Dr. Frank Weinstock's writings are so relevant. The next best thing to having a trusted

Praise For *I've Been Thinking*
By Frank J. Weinstock, M.D., F.A.C.S.

physician with whom we can just sit and talk about our questions, is having Dr. Weinstock's book at our disposal. Writing in a direct, easily understood manner, while avoiding unnecessary medical jargon, Dr. Weinstock conveys to the reader a confidence that 'this guy knows what he's talking about!' Finding trustworthy information about our health questions can relieve our anxieties and give us a sense of personal control. So I recommend this book, not only to patients who want practical answers to their questions, but also to practicing physicians and other health care professionals who would like not only to enhance their 'bedside manners' but also to be able to communicate more effectively and empathetically with their patients."

—Ted Strickland, Ph.D., *Ex-Governor*
  State of Ohio

Praise For *I've Been Thinking*
By Frank J. Weinstock, M.D., F.A.C.S.

"Who hasn't asked the question, 'Am I paying too much for health care?' If you are like me, you have also likely complained about the complexities of health insurance plans. Well, those days may be over. Dr. Frank Weinstock has written a handy and helpful book that answers a wide array of questions about health care. From emergency room visits, to Medicare benefits, to when to replace your glasses, Weinstock's book has the answer. Readers will find this practical guide both easy to understand and chock-full of straightforward advice. I wholeheartedly recommend it to you!"

—Robert P. Watson, Ph.D., *Professor of American Studies Lynn University*

"Finally . . . a book that helps the average consumer make sound health care decisions among the myriad of choices, plans and options available in the increasingly complex health environment. Dr. Frank Weinstock is a noted, board-certified ophthalmologist and longtime health care management consultant. A must-read for everyone who wants to make wise decisions related to health care and value."

—Para Jones, Ph.D., *President Stark State College (Canton, OH)*

Praise For *I've Been Thinking*
By Frank J. Weinstock, M.D., F.A.C.S.

"Frank Weinstock, M.D., noted ophthalmologist, lecturer and columnist, has distilled fifty years of experience as an expert provider and advisor into a concise patient handbook, written in the same breezy style that made his columns so popular. Dr. Weinstock devotes the first half of his book to both education and critical self-advocacy for patients facing the complicated morass that is today's health care system. In the remaining chapters, he focuses on his own specialty, the eye, and the bewildering array of diseases, procedures and appliances that so many of us encounter. For patients and their family members, this book provides an important opportunity to re-examine their role not as passive consumers of health care, but as active participants and advocates."

—Rob Crane, M.D., *Clinical Associate Professor*
  The Ohio State University

"Probably the single most problem that faces all of us is our personal health. Dr. Frank Weinstock's book offers clear and complete answers."

—Michael Dann, *Former Vice-President of Programming*
  C.B.S.

I'VE BEEN THINKING

AND IT MIGHT SAVE YOUR LIFE (AND VISION)

FRANK J. WEINSTOCK, M.D., F.A.C.S.

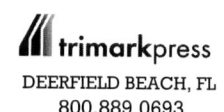

DEERFIELD BEACH, FL
800.889.0693

Copyright ©2014 by Frank J. Weinstock, M.D., F.A.C.S.
All rights reserved.

No part of this publication may be reproduced or transmitted in any form or by any means, electronic, mechanical or otherwise, including photocopy, recording, or any information storage or retrieval system now known or to be invented, without permission in writing from the publisher, except by a reviewer who wishes to quote brief passages in connection with a review. Requests for permission should be addressed in writing to the publisher—publisher@trimarkpress.com.

Limit of Liability/Disclaimer of Warranty: While the publisher and author have used their best efforts in preparing this book, they make no representations or warranties with respect to the accuracy or completeness of the contents of this book and specifically disclaim any implied warranties of merchantability or fitness for a particular purpose.

Library of Congress Cataloging-in-Publication Data

I've Been Thinking... And it Might Save Your Life and Vision

Frank J. Weinstock, M.D., F.A.C.S.

p. cm.

ISBN: 978-0-9886145-9-8
Library of Congress Control Number:

A14

10 9 8 7 6 5 4 3 2 1

First Edition

Printed and Bound in the United States of America

www.DrFrankWeinstock.com

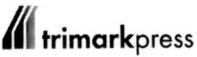

A Publication of TriMark Press, Inc.
368 South Military Trail
Deerfield Beach, FL 33442
800.889.0693
www.TriMarkPress.com

Dedication

Family is what makes everything worthwhile, and I wish to dedicate this book to my support system:

My wife, Saragale.

My children, their spouses and (their children):

Michael and Beth Weinstock
(Olivia, Eli, Theo and Annie)

Jill and Ted Deutch
(Gabrielle, Serena and Cole)

Jeffrey and Lillian Weinstock
(Ryan and Kyle)

I also want to thank my many patients, who over the years have taught me much about life and how to deal with it.

Acknowledgments

Several people were instrumental in my preparing this book. First, my wife and children critically evaluated this work and gave me much encouragement.

John Johnson, my former editor at the *Boca News*, is one of my best supporters and provided excellent guidance and editing. His encouragement was invaluable in my arriving at the point of publication. Barry Chesler, publisher of TriMark Press, and Penelope Love, publishing director, also have been extremely helpful in the entire publishing process, making it as seamless as possible.

Having written medical columns for years, I appreciate the positive comments and reinforcement that friends and readers have given me.

TABLE OF CONTENTS

Preface . . . xix

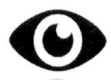

Section 1: A Peek

1
It's No Longer Your Grandparents' Hospital Or Doctor's Office . . . 1

2
How Do I Find Good Medical Care? . . . 5

3
The Chaos And Confusion In The Practice Of Medicine . . . 9

4
Choosing A Physician . . . 13

5
Emergency Departments . . . 17

6
Hospital Emergency Rooms . . . 21

TABLE OF CONTENTS

7
Expectations And Questions—Or When To Say More Than *"Ahhhh"* ... 29

8
Continuing With "It's More Than Just Saying 'Ahhhh'" ... 37

9
Medicine—An Art Or A Science? ... 43

10
Medicare Can Be A Muddle ... 47

11
Medical Costs—How Do You Know? ... 57

12
So You Think You're Paying Too Much? ... 63

13
The Reality And The Myth Of Prevention ... 69

14
What Was That Again? ... 75

15
Talked With Any Patients Lately? ... 79

16
Management Of Lab Results— A Fly In Your Ointment ... 83

TABLE OF CONTENTS

17
Huh? . . . 87

18
If You Don't Ask You Won't Know . . . 93

19
Electronic Medical Records—A Salvation Or A Salve? . . . 97

20
There Are Potholes On The Quality Care Road—Ask . . . 101

21
Unhappy With The Doc? What Do You Do? . . . 103

22
Still Unhappy? More Thoughts. . . . 107

23
Medicine For All—Telemedicine . . . 111

24
Medicine For All—Telemedicine's Future . . . 115

Section 2: More Than A Glance

25
But It's Just Routine—Right? . . . 121

26
Whose Health Is It Anyway? . . . 125

TABLE OF CONTENTS

27
Eye Problems And The Specialists . . . 131

28
Can My Child's Crossed Eyes Be Outgrown? . . . 137

29
Can Near-Sightedness Progression Be Stopped? . . . 141

30
Glasses, Glasses—The Differences Are Many . . . 145

31
Don't Like Glasses?
There Are Choices Beyond Contacts . . . 153

32
I'm Having Trouble With My Glasses or Contacts. Why? . . . 159

33
How Often Should I Have My Glasses Changed? . . . 165

34
Taking Your Contacts On Vacation . . . 169

35
Botox Has More Uses Than Mere Vanity . . . 173

36
Contact Lenses—Also Not Merely For Vanity . . . 177

37
Diabetes And The Eye—Your Role . . . 183

TABLE OF CONTENTS

38
Most People Have Cataracts? . . . 189

39
On The Other Side of the Scalpel . . . 193

40
Your Doctor Doesn't Have X-Ray Vision . . . 201

41
The Second Opinion—Wait A Second! . . . 207

42
Second Opinions—A Few Seconds More . . . 211

43
So What's An Advocate? . . . 215

44
What Hand Am I Holding Up, Doc? . . . 219

45
What Constitutes An Eye Emergency? . . . 225

46
What Should I Look For In
An Eye Exam? . . . 229

47
Aging And Your Eyes . . . 233

48
Falling—And Not In Love . . . 239

TABLE OF CONTENTS

49
Having Trouble Driving At Night? . . . 245

50
You Want To Celebrate Having An Eye Injury? . . . 249

51
What Is Vision Screening? . . . 251

52
What Determines The Color Of Eyes? . . . 253

53
Lasers Are More Than Science Fiction . . . 255

54
You Wanna Cut What? . . . 259

55
Seniors See Better Without Glasses—
"Second Sight?" . . . 263

Section 3: Flat Out Staring

56
Cataract Surgery—A Matter Of New Lenses . . . 267

57
Macular Degeneration—Is There Hope? . . . 271

TABLE OF CONTENTS

58
What's "Lazy Eye" And How Is It Treated? . . . 277

59
A Vitreous What? . . . 279

60
What's That Floating In My Eye? . . . 281

61
Why Do My Eyes Water A Lot? . . . 287

62
Will Ultraviolet Light Harm The Eyes? . . . 291

63
Strokes Can And Do Affect The Eyes . . . 293

64
Thyroid Disease And Your Eyes . . . 295

65
Hey—You Have One Pupil Larger! . . . 297

66
Retinitis Pigmentosa—Smaller And Smaller And Smaller . . . 301

67
I'm Not Sleepy—I Just Have Ptosis . . . 305

68
Eye Drops and You . . . 307

TABLE OF CONTENTS

69
How Does Herpes Simplex Affect
The Eye? ... 309

70
Can Juvenile Arthritis Affect The Eyes? ... 313

71
What's "Pressure" In The Eye? ... 315

72
Can AIDS Affect The Eye? ... 319

Afterword ... 321

About the Author ... 322

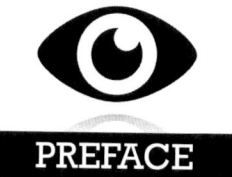

PREFACE

While the health care system is changing rapidly, patient needs are not changing—and thus guidance is useful and often needed. The ultimate goal for you is to maximize system benefits while avoiding misdiagnosis and extraneous testing. This book can prevent much aggravation and misunderstanding when dealing with the "system"—and it could also save your life.

Medicine is no longer the bedside experience your grandparents received. After the office evaluation by a physician or other provider, patients are often left alone to deal with issues of reimbursement, co-payments, deductibles, referrals, medication side effects, and if necessary, a surgical procedure or hospital stay. This book shows ways to deal with these concerns—and also why and how patients can and *must* be active health care participants.

Writing monthly newspaper columns, along with lectures to lay and professional groups, has given the author many insights. This book shares those insights and reveals the surprising inner workings of a disorienting health care network—insights learned both as a physician and as a patient.

And with sight loss being one of the most feared health losses, the author also discusses a number of eye conditions and some of the amazing eye health and help options available. These conditions range from children's vision problems to "lazy" eye and glasses as well as cataracts, retinal diseases and low vision.

As patients, we deserve the best care available—and while it's a common attitude that we should not question our doctor's edicts, the author's recommendations are different. To receive the best care, patients *must* understand how physicians think and how the medical system works. This book lays those secrets bare and outlines a strategy for health care success.

SECTION 1

A Peek

CHAPTER 1

It's No Longer Your Grandparents' Hospital Or Doctor's Office

It's confusing. Gone are the days of the family doctor providing birth to death care in the office. Gone are the days when your family doctor managed your illness when you went to the hospital.

Now, there are many different people who participate in your care. Often it's difficult to tell them apart! In your grandparents' hospital, nurses wore hats, which were distinctive as to the school each attended. In your grandparents' hospital, physicians wore long, white coats and introduced themselves as Doctor. In your grandparents' hospital, medical students, interns and residents often wore short, white coats. Today, many physicians do not wear jackets or ties (actually it has been shown that ties may be the source of some infections). Today, many physicians come to the office or hospital in jeans. There's no longer a uniform by which you can tell who's who. It's important for you to ask the role of those with whom you come in contact.

A *New York Times* article dealt with the use of the term "Doctor" in hospitals and medical offices, as many institutions now have a doctorate in nursing. This might be confusing, especially if you're a new patient in an office or the hospital and don't know the physician you're supposed to see. Stereotypically, we are used to seeing male physicians wearing white coats; with male nurses it may be more confusing. Nonetheless, it's your job to know who's seeing you. If you're in the hospital or a doctor's office, there's nothing wrong with asking the individual where he or she fits in.

In order to run an office efficiently there is extensive us of ancillary personnel who have specific roles, such as measuring and recording vital signs, drawing blood, and performing special testing. Using ancillary personnel allows the physician to offer more services than would be impossible without them.

For example, in our ophthalmology office we can provide extensive glaucoma testing, photography of the eye, various types of laser treatments and much more. Ancillary personnel are used for inputting your most recent history and medications into the computer for physician review. The most efficient office will utilize every resource available to gather accurate data on which the physician can base his or her diagnostic decisions.

There are also mid-level providers (MLP's), including physician assistants and nurse practitioners that may independently perform the history and exam and prescribe the treatment. Just as when there is a concern with the physician's management of your condition, if there is a concern about the mid-level provider, it's an option to discuss your management with the supervising physician.

Differentiating the staff in your own doctor's office is difficult enough, but this task is compounded exponentially in the hospital, where multiple providers are involved, multiple shifts are utilized, and personnel enter and exit your room repeatedly. Again, don't be afraid to ask who someone is and where he or she fits in. There should be one physician, usually a primary care doctor or hospitalist, managing your entire care.

If you're going to surgery, you may ask who's going to do the surgery and who's going to be in the operating room. Especially in teaching centers, the surgery may be carried out completely by a physician in training. There is nothing inherently wrong with this, but you should know the situation and discuss this with your surgeon, preferably before you go to the hospital. And with the increasing use of "hospitalists"—doctors who are hospital based rather than in a private office—you might not even see your primary physician after you go to the hospital. When used correctly and efficiently, ancillary personnel in the office and hospital are of great benefit to the patient and to the physician, more confusing than your grandparents' hospital, but hopefully more efficient.

CHAPTER 2

How Do I Find Good Medical Care?

There are several factors that control the ability to get high quality medical care. The two most important are availability of care and affordability of care.

Availability of good quality care varies tremendously. In many ways it's proportional to the number of physicians and hospitals. Care is definitely limited without them. Although most problems may be handled by a good primary care physician, the need for specialists and super specialists may be necessary. If you are in smaller remote areas, they may not be available or accessible. With modern transportation, this is less of a problem than in the past, but time and distance can be critical in an emergency and also may be prohibitive for an ill individual needing special diagnostic and treatment facilities.

Larger metropolitan areas have a wealth of expertise in physicians and hospitals, including specialists and super-specialists.

How do you choose a physician? This is more difficult than one would expect. Many of the "best" physicians have great communication skills and large practices, but they may be short on expertise. Probably the only way you will know definitively how good your physician is would be in a crisis situation when the skill will be readily apparent. Ideally you will want a physician whose personality meshes with yours.

However, the best recommendation may be from another physician (either a local physician or, if you are in a new community, the physician you saw in the past. If we don't know a physician elsewhere personally, we can look up physicians and their qualifications in directories. Recognize that much of the information in directories may actually be advertisements, paid by the physician.

Hospitals and medical societies have referral services, but these will often recommend the "next" physician "in line" without any real knowledge about his or her qualifications.

After you get one or several names, you can ask friends about their experiences or look him or her up online. The office site will obviously be complimentary, but will give biased information as to his or her qualifications and the services provided by the office. Friends can give information that may be very valuable since they may be going to that physician and may have done a certain amount of investigation first themselves.

Online sites may give information as to malpractice claims and possible disciplinary actions by the state medical board.

A simple call to the office asking about the physician's qualifications, such as specialty areas, board certification, hospital affiliations, etc., will give you information as to how the office responds to patients and how patients are treated.

After all of this investigation, it may be very frustrating to have to make a choice, only to be told by the office staff that they are not taking new patients. Try to have several names in case this happens.

CHAPTER 3

The Chaos And Confusion In The Practice Of Medicine

In general, the practice of medicine is more exciting and more gratifying than ever before. The increased longevity and improved lifestyle of patients is proof that we are making diagnoses and successfully treating conditions that were never possible to treat in the past. With microscopes, gene therapy, DNA discoveries, the ability to grow new limbs, etc., it's exciting to wake up almost every day to new advances.

Then why is there so much apparent dissatisfaction by physicians with the work each has chosen to do?

As has the world in general, the field of medicine has undergone rapid technological, social and economic change—and there's a natural human tendency to be fearful of change. Many younger physicians, such as my son, in emergency medicine tell me that the "new" field of medicine is not a great problem because now is now, and thus what was different in the past is not known to current practitioners.

However, there's much opposition to the current state of medical affairs from physicians who have been in practice for a number of years. These professionals yearn for the "good old days" when the physician was "king" and had the ultimate control of all aspects of medicine. These doctors often complain about current fee structures, stressing that physician income is regulated and not what it was in the past. Hopefully, these doctors went into the medical field because of the patient and not just the resulting income. At the same time, it's a reality that third party insurance payments, government regulations, and paperwork in general have increased the frustration and decreased the satisfaction of physicians.

Physicians are individuals who often have strong opinions about most things. When it comes to the diagnosis and management of patients, interference is resented. It interferes with us carrying out our role as physicians and often may be detrimental to patient care, since cost is often the most important factor in many third party insurance company decisions. Recognizing that medical costs have escalated tremendously, it's often mentioned that a fee-for-service concept encourages poor medicine, unnecessary surgery, etc. This may occur and should be eliminated by strict oversight and prosecution when it's discovered.

In many ways, private practice should be economical since physicians have no need to boost revenues by ordering many tests and procedures to keep his or her employer happy. This is changing with increased emphasis on practicing quality medicine and only ordering tests and procedures when truly indicated.

However, the alternative of placing physicians on a salary does not ensure quality of care nor a reduction in unnecessary procedures. Having worked in and observed many situations where physicians are on strict salary, I have noticed problems. Many excellent physicians are in salaried positions, however the need for power more than income can result in producing poor medical care. Unnecessary surgery, excess costs, and lack of concern for individual patients may result from the quest for power. Keeping patients in the hospital longer than necessary may assure a greater budget or more beds for the next fiscal year. This is nothing new. Carrying out more surgery may result in increased revenues in time for the physician and the employer.

A good physician will practice high quality medicine regardless of where he or she practices. With physicians having many different personalities, there are many different types of practice from which to choose.

There are no simple answers for the problems of medicine in the current age. There's no question, however, that the major concern of physicians should remain the provision of excellent care for all individuals. Third-party payors and the government should provide appropriate oversight. Rapid advances in all aspects of medicine make the practice of medicine more exciting every day.

CHAPTER 4

Choosing A Physician

It's usually best to have a primary care physician who does the initial evaluation since it's often not necessary to see a specialist. This may save much time and testing. If referral is necessary your primary care physician may make this process much smoother and efficient.

When there are known specific problems such as orthopedic, cardiac, eye, etc., you should have a relationship with these specialists.

This is especially important to those who get their primary medical care elsewhere such as retired persons or those who vacation away from their hometown. In these situations, you still need local physicians in case of an emergency.

There is increasing use of concierge physicians, whereby you pay an up-front fee (usually between $1,000-$2,000) for care in a practice which sees many fewer patients and is always available for care. These practices can refer you much more quickly and efficiently than most standard practices. Patients who use concierge practices appear to be extremely happy and feel that the added expense is worth it.

Apparently many physicians do not see emergencies in their office and automatically tell patients that, "if you think this is an emergency, go to the nearest emergency room." Because of this, many patients simply go there themselves without even calling the office. This results in higher expenses.

In emergency situations, emergency rooms vary in their capabilities and services. The ability of a facility to handle your emergency may vary significantly. There are sophisticated emergency departments that can handle almost any emergency as contrasted with smaller facilities that may have only one room and a physician on call with minimal sophisticated emergency equipment. Know your insurance since it may not cover emergency visits if it is not a true emergency.

Primary care is now being offered in pharmacies and superstores, which may employ physician assistants or nurse practitioners to provide limited care. They can handle many health problems and will refer you to physicians when necessary. You should be informed and choose the care that is appropriate for your problem.

In choosing physicians, hospitals, or any type of medical care, you may want to check the Internet for more information or ratings. Be aware that much information on the Internet is paid advertising. There are many rating sites that must be evaluated by you as to their accuracy.

CHAPTER 5

Emergency Departments

Emergency departments vary in their ability to handle problems and are classified according to their ability to handle more serious problems. Some are more sophisticated and may specialize in orthopedics, cardiac, pediatric or neurological problems, etc. If the paramedics are involved, they do an initial evaluation and will determine where to take you for your care. They often consult with the emergency department via phone and usually take the patient to the nearest hospital, unless they know that specialized care is necessary elsewhere.

In larger areas, when you are seen in the emergency room, you will be examined by ancillary personnel or the physician on duty who, hopefully, will be a trained emergency room physician. In many areas, it may be a physician who left his or her primary care practice to work in the emergency room for any number of reasons. Increasingly you may be cared for by a nurse practitioner or a physician's assistant who is trained in diagnosis, treatment and suturing, usually under the supervision of a physician. These professionals are very capable and often decrease your time in the emergency department significantly while allowing the physician to handle the more complicated problems.

If you require additional care or referral, such as orthopedic, ophthalmological, cardiac or other specialties, they usually call the specialist on call. In these situations, as well as others, you may want to discuss this beforehand and you may want to discuss the physician who is being called and decide if you want this physician or want to call your own.

You may want to call your personal physician to ask for advice before using the referral physician who is on call for the emergency room.

In actuality, unless you are going to the hospital on your own, you do not have much choice of which hospital to use.

Be aware of your insurance, which may limit your emergency care. If you are taken to a hospital with physicians who are not on your plan, there may be a problem having your insurance company pay for the care or physicians. There are situations in which the insurance company may feel that it wasn't necessary to go to the emergency department and will not pay the bill. Many facilities now advertise their "wait times" on the Internet, or on billboards on a highway or near the hospital.

It's very frustrating to be sick and have a long wait in the emergency department. Another choice is to go to an urgent care center. These are staffed by trained urgent care physicians who handle or manage many problems. They are not usually equipped to handle life-threatening emergencies but can manage many problems that require care, but are not life threatening. They are usually independent facilities and not a part of the hospital such as is the emergency department. They are a useful addition when you feel you need care and your physician is not available.

You should think about potential health emergencies and have a plan written out for yourself or your family to follow. This should include your medical history, your medications, the names and phone numbers of your physicians, the name of your preferred emergency room and who is authorized to receive information from the physicians so that the emergency room or urgent care staff can discuss your situation since they cannot discuss your health with anyone else unless they have your specific consent.

Pharmacies and superstores are now being staffed with nurse practitioners or physician assistants who act independenly and are able to handle many less extensive medical situations.

CHAPTER 6

Hospital Emergency Rooms

For a number of reasons you may find yourself in an emergency room—what should you know beforehand?

It may be that you or a family member had chest pain or an injury; you may have a cold and don't want to go to your doctor; you might not have a doctor; you may have fallen and gotten hurt.

First, you should have a plan so that you and your family know which emergency room is your preference if the occasion arrives.

You must decide whether or not to go to an emergency room. Your insurance company may have guidelines, especially mentioning the company's preferred emergency facility. The company might not cover your expenses if you go to another emergency room.

We hate to admit it but it should be mentioned that men are somewhat unreliable, tending to minimize their health—often delaying the care until problems have occurred. This means women (spouses, etc.) must frequently take the initiative to direct us males to seek medical help.

When you have an urgent situation, some decisions must be made. As a physician, I like patients to call me first for a decision as to where to go. In general, if possible, many physicians prefer to see the patient in the office since we have much specialized equipment that may not be available in the hospital. Seeing you in the office may also be a major cost-saving measure. However, for heart attacks, strokes and other acute conditions, the hospital is the place to be.

If possible, call your physician if you don't know what to do. If there is unrelieved chest pain, unexpected and unrelieved shortness of breath on exertion, uncontrollable bleeding, disorientation or confusion, difficult trauma or feeling that the situation is out of control, you should consider going to the emergency room. If you need specialized experience or equipment, or if you can't be moved, you should consider calling 911 for transportation. Otherwise you might want to go by car, which might be faster, but more dangerous since required emergency care might be delayed. The type of care you receive will be the same whether you arrive by private car or ambulance. Some people feel that, if they arrive in an ambulance, even for minor conditions, they will get faster care. In major trauma, they talk of the "Golden Hour," which means that treatment is essential in the first hour in order to survive. So don't delay in an emergency situation.

If the paramedics are called, they will have continual contact with the emergency room for advice and to let the emergency room know that they are on the way. Sadly, occasionally your insurance carrier will make a determination that, in their opinion, your situation was not urgent and should not be covered by your policy.

Whoever arrives at the emergency room, whether by ambulance or as a walk-in, is met by a triage (sorting) nurse who will ask some questions to initially determine the type of care needed and the urgency. It's essential to try to determine who is sickest and needs the most immediate care first. You must recognize that, in spite of your discomfort, there may be patients who are more seriously ill and must be cared for first. Be understanding and be tolerant of the staff.

If you are in the ER with a patient (whether a spouse or a friend), you will not be able to stay with the patient unless he or she gives specific permission. When you are with the patient, it's important that you do not leave the bedside to "wander" around since this may interfere with someone else's care. Another reason that you will not be allowed to walk around is because each person's privacy must be protected. With a family member, have a signed permission slip that might allow you to communicate with the staff about his or her condition. Once you are assigned to a bed, multiple people, including the physician, will ask you questions, often the same as the previous person. This is essential to verify the facts and to arrive at a correct diagnosis.

Recognize that, on a national basis, about 80 percent of the people seen in emergency rooms are not emergencies. Because of this, some insurance companies may not pay for non-emergency care if you go to the ER. However, if you feel it's an emergency, you should be there to be evaluated.

Patients are admitted on an as-needed basis. It doesn't matter if they come by ambulance or walk in. A preliminary triage series of questions determines where they go and how soon they receive care. Ability to pay is not an issue. It's interesting that the cost of care for many non-paying patients is absorbed by the hospitals—they may not receive compensation from the state or federal government for these expenses. In some areas of the country, a large number of uninsured, non-paying patients will cause a financial hardship for the hospital.

Some emergency room areas provide information as to the length of wait time. This might be on a billboard or require you to call a number at the hospital. The emergency room is a busy place. Since sicker people are given priority, there may be a significant wait for minor problems. The hospital ER should not be used for convenience or after hours care for minor conditions.

At the hospital, there may be are three parts of the emergency process to which a patient is assigned after being seen by the triage individual. Interestingly, the triage and assignment are carried out first with no questions regarding insurance or ability to pay. Federal law (EMTALA) prohibits emergency rooms to refuse treatment or divert patients who may be unable to pay. However, without insurance, you will eventually be charged at the highest rates available. This is not logical, but it's the law. There are emergency care centers (actually urgent care centers or hospital emergency facilities for the management of minor injuries, colds, etc.

The emergency department will first handle those patients who have a true emergency and may need special care for their problems. There is a staff of emergency physicians (most, if not all, board certified) who will administer care. The hospital staff of specialists is available on call for specialty care such as eyes, ears, orthopedics, etc.

In certain situations that cannot be handled and require super specialized care, e.g., neurosurgical care, heart surgery, etc. the patient might require referral to a facility where this care is available. It's important that the patient be stabilized first before transporting him or her elsewhere. Many hospitals have an open heart surgery unit (for bypass or stent surgery). Patients requiring special expertise have to be transported to hospitals that handle that type of problem.

However in the event of an emergency, the patient should be transported to the nearest facility for stabilization and evaluation of the specifics of his or her condition. In cardiac situations, the hospitals may be prepared to administer clot busters (anticoagulants) and stabilize patients, with referral if indicated. If further care such as by-pass surgery is indicated, at this time such patients will have to be transported to special hospitals that deal with these problems.

There is a third group of patients that passes through the emergency room as "direct admissions." These are patients who are sent to the hospital by their private physicians for admission, but do not actually require the staff of the emergency room.

As far as costs go, it's usually more expensive to go to the emergency room. Some insurance policies say that you won't be covered if it's not an emergency. If you feel it's an emergency, do not try to figure out if your insurance will cover the costs. In disputes, it's usually settled in favor of the patient if the patient feels that the situation is truly an emergency.

CHAPTER 7

Expectations And Questions —Or When To Say More Than *"Ahhhh"*

Many people complain about doctors in general. I believe much of this discontent is created by poor communication from the doctor and/or staff and, occasionally, somewhat unrealistic expectations from the patient.

How do you decide which physician should care for you? Often it's a friend or neighbor who makes the recommendation. If you have been going to a physician in your city (or in another city), ask him or her for a recommendation. Beware of fancy ads and web sites. They may provide interesting information, but make sure to find out if it is accurate and correct.

What's the minimum to expect?

- A caring physician and staff.
- Courtesy from everyone involved.
- Answers to questions and concerns.
- Notification of test results in a timely manner.

Of course, the most important aspects of care are the correct diagnosis and treatment. This means that there must be communication between the physician and the patient—and remember that it's a two-way street.

When we deal with babies, the communication is more by observation and listening to the reaction of the child. The older patient must convey his or her concerns to the physician and the physician must communicate by asking for information.

What should you do if you feel your needs are not being met?

The first thing is to discuss any concerns with the physician. This will usually resolve your concerns. In my opinion, a small number of physicians enjoy the practice of medicine, but do not like talking with patients. Also, some don't want to get involved with how the office and practice are run. He or she may be totally unaware of your concerns and that "the office" is not following through in providing the service that should be standard. If, and after communicating your concerns the physician is not interested or does not answer your questions adequately, the answer is simple—ask for your records and go elsewhere. Before asking for your records, make sure that you are accepted at another practice.

In any case, there are several specific areas that should be dealt with up front when going to any physician. Before you go to the office, understand your financial obligation:

- Does the physician accept Medicare or other insurance?
- What will your obligation otherwise be?

Some physicians require total payment first and expect the patient to handle the insurance. In general, if Medicare does not cover a procedure, the physician must notify you in advance and get written permission from you agreeing to the procedure and its cost. If not notified in advance, the doctor is not allowed to charge you for the procedure. If a participating Medicare provider performs a service or procedure, he must accept what Medicare pays without charging you any more than this payment.

The diagnosis or the plan to make a diagnosis (often an answer to your problems is not found on the first exam) should also be discussed up front so that you know what's happening. The findings on the exam and the plan for the future should then be clarified periodically.

If tests or medications are prescribed, each should be explained. If a test is performed or if a biopsy is taken, how long will it be before you can expect to hear about the results? Prescriptions should be explained with written instructions, when indicated. If you're taking medications, each should be written down with specific instructions as to dosage and timing. Potential side effects, within reason, should be mentioned or written out (this is often done by the pharmacist).

Other issues that you should learn about up front include:

- What happens if you need after-hours care or simply have questions?

- Is your physician available or is it necessary to go to an emergency room?
- Are there other physicians in the practice, or does your doctor share call with other offices?
- In case of questions or an emergency, will the physician be available or how will these situations be handled?

There's almost nothing without risk. Especially with surgery, invasive testing and surgery, the indications, risks and alternatives of the test or surgery must be discussed, giving you a chance to ask questions. Likewise, there's also nothing wrong with inquiring about the experience of a physician or hospital, for instance:

- Has he performed this procedure before?
- What's his complication rate?
- If a new procedure, how many has he performed?
- Is this the best hospital for the procedure?
- If being sent to a hospital for surgery, what's the infection rate?
- How often is this procedure done at that hospital?

- What's the mortality rate?
- Especially with catheters, what's the hospital infection rate compared with others?

Much of this comparative information is available on the Internet, i.e., disciplinary actions against physicians, hospital performance in a number of categories, etc.

Other questions:

- If you're having surgery, will your physician perform the procedure or will a resident or fellow be allowed to perform the surgery?
- Will students be in the operating room; if so, what will their role be?

If a procedure is recommended to be performed in the physician's office or an ambulatory center, inquire about the safety, the facilities, how an emergency might be handled, who will be giving anesthesia, have there been deaths after an anticipated minor procedure and ask anything else that might concern you.

If you're not recovering from a condition or doing well after surgery, there's nothing wrong with seeking a second opinion. When getting a second opinion, it's best to do it with the help of your physician. He or she can make an appointment for you and provide the background information, which will make your appointment more efficient since it will eliminate testing and repetition of procedures. Fortunately, it's unusual to find differences of opinion in most situations, but it may be significant in some rare situations and life-saving in others.

Obviously many points were made above and it would not be practical to go over all of them in a short visit. Inquire about the most important things first and go into the others when appropriate. Some physicians may resent you asking many of these questions. If so, you may want to seek care elsewhere.

Fortunately, in my experience, most physicians practice good medicine, are dedicated to taking the best care of patients, and are happy to answer questions. It's rare to come up with a problem situation. The bottom line is that obtaining quality medical care requires communication between the physician and patients in order to obtain the best results.

CHAPTER 8

Continuing With "It's More Than Just Saying '*Ahhhh*'"

As noted in the last chapter, communication is a two-way street and you need to make sure your side of that street is well-paved with good intentions—and a smile. On the other side of the street, some complaints about physicians may be justified, for instance:

- Not calling with results of laboratory tests
- Not returning phone calls
- Impolite office staff, etc.

Quite often, there's a misunderstanding that has not been brought to the doctor's attention.

Fortunately, this applies to only a minority of doctors, but it shouldn't happen at all. Adequate two-way communication is unquestionably beneficial and necessary to your health. The questions asked by the physician and patient, as well as the answers and explanations, are essential to arriving at the correct diagnosis and treatment.

As with all of us, physicians may communicate in either a more or less effective manner. If your physician is not communicating in the manner that you expect, it's almost always unintentional and requires that we communicate any problems. Doctors also respond to us negatively if we, as patients, aren't nice, overly demanding—or just plain rude. In these cases the physician may respond in a negative manner—as likely would anyone.

When dealing with a physician, it's important to be pleasant and friendly. Don't be afraid to smile and say things such as, "How are you doing, doctor?" Wear a smile, since this is often contagious. The patient is often stressed out with his or her problem and the physician may be stressed with his or her own problems as well. This must be recognized and then left out of the interaction on both sides of the street.

When you have concerns, usually accumulated

over a period of time, write them down with the date of your problem, how it has affected you, how long has it lasted, anything that made it better, etc. This is much more accurate and efficient than trying to recall it under the pressure of the office visit.

If you don't understand things, don't be afraid to ask for explanations and to ask for written instructions, such as:

- Which medications to take?
- How often?
- What are the side effects?
- What's the prognosis, etc.?

As physicians, we always feel that we're communicating well, but need your help when it isn't clear to you. When starting with a new physician, discuss with him and/or the staff what you should expect. For example:

- Some physicians will tell you that they always return phone calls, or instead that the staff returns the calls—ask.
- Some physicians will tell you to not expect a call about laboratory tests or pathology unless there's a problem.

- Find out how long it will take to be seen if you have a routine problem or an emergency. Some offices have enough physicians to provide coverage all the time, whereas others may tell you to go to the emergency room routinely if you have a problem.

- If you're going to a solo practitioner (one who has no other physicians or partners in the office), find out how you will obtain care after hours, or if he's on vacation.

Sometimes there's bad chemistry, but often this may be corrected with adequate communication. If you're unhappy with the answers, this is the time to recognize it and seek medical care elsewhere. If there's a problem in the office or with the physician, it's essential to verbalize it. Physicians are often oblivious about what's going on in the office, preferring to concentrate on medicine rather than office beauty or atmosphere.

If staff is impolite or inefficient, the physician should be notified about it since he or she may not see this aspect of the office. The same applies to staff attitudes—and also applies to how the staff responds or talks to patients, whether on the phone or in the office. On your side of the street, be generous with compliments to the physician and the staff—both appreciate it.

Most physicians are interested and can only correct problems if told about them. Although problems should be obvious to the staff, there are many instances in which a patient must bring up the topic. If you mention problems, it should be done in a professional, non-threatening way. Otherwise, an untenable, antagonistic situation might arise. If the physician is not interested in a problem or makes excuses that aren't valid, it might be necessary to seek care elsewhere.

Fortunately, most physicians are interested in maintaining a pleasant, efficient office, although there are exceptions. Poor communication between you and your physician in an inefficient office is frustrating and may be detrimental to your health.

CHAPTER 9

Medicine—An Art Or A Science?

Modern medicine has made great strides in the development of a multitude of diagnostic tests: X-rays, blood tests, CAT scans, MRI's, ultrasound and many more. We often joke that all we have to do is put the patient into a machine—making the physician expendable. Nevertheless, it's not unusual for a physician to order a battery of tests before seeing the patient, hoping that one of them might provide an answer before examining the patient or asking any questions. With certain medical conditions, it's helpful for the physician to have these results available before or at the time of the exam.

Usually, the physician will see the results of these tests before your exam and discuss them with you. Since they occasionally may be missed, don't be afraid to bring up the topic and ask for the results of the testing.

The results of many of these tests are available to the physician within hours. Obviously the physician must review them, which may take some time and requires that this time be fit into an already busy schedule. Either way the patient, who's often anxious, should be notified about the results as soon as possible.

On the other hand, as patients we should be reasonable and not be in a rush to get results of routine tests, which may be important but aren't critical. However, if a reasonable time has elapsed and you haven't heard from the office, don't be afraid to call. Sometimes reports are misfiled and your call will remind everyone that you haven't been notified.

What's the purpose of testing? It should be used to confirm or make diagnoses and should be customized to the patient, along with following the progress of a disease and determining the necessary treatment.

There are legitimate screening tests, as well as

tests such as those for diabetes, high blood pressure, breast cancer, etc. Testing may have a purpose of confirming symptoms or suspicions. The days of simply ordering every test available are gone; testing must have a purpose.

A few years ago there was a lot of advertising, mainly from hospitals and other owners of CAT scan machines, to get whole body scans in search of something bad. Although it sounds great, and in spite of picking up some issues, much harm was done. As a result of some vague shadow on these exams it was not unusual for patients to undergo serious operations even though no disease was found. In fact, some patients developed complications or died from the resulting surgery.

This isn't to say disease was *never* found. It was the feeling, however, that, at best, psychological harm occurred to many patients because of these false positives and that more harm than good may result from "shotgun" testing.

Obviously we would like to pick up all disease, but this isn't possible. Still, patients are reassured by testing and are often responsible for pushing the physician to order tests that might not be indicated. This is often seen with CAT scans and MRI's, especially with minor head injuries in children, thereby exposing the child to unnecessary radiation and false positives. The physician's goal is to see the patient, take a careful history, compare this exam with past findings, and order the tests that are indicated. This is the art of medicine, in which the physician's part is still the most important aspect of an exam.

Screening exams such as those for colon cancer, diabetes, glaucoma, and many other diseases are indicated and should be carried out as suggested by your physician.

We want to perform the minimum amount of testing in order to provide the best care to the patient. Even though insurance and Medicare pays for most testing, we should be cautious about requiring tests so that the system can be affordable for everyone. We all need to recognize that testing may be harmful and may be extremely expensive to the system and to the patient. Tests are in fact only an addition to the physician's exam—as he or she practices the art of medicine.

CHAPTER 10

Medicare Can Be A Muddle

Who's your insurance carrier? If you have Medicare, is it sold through a company, hospital, or other entity? Do you have a contact person in case you have questions about your health insurance? Do you need to get prior authorization for certain tests or procedures? This is often required for cosmetic and expensive surgical procedures or treatments. Are you limited to certain physicians, hospitals or facilities for testing and care? Is it required that the company must give permission before the service is carried out or it will not pay for the service, meaning that you will be responsible? This is primarily for cosmetic procedures, but may be required for almost any type of procedure, test or simply for any office visit, especially if they are very expensive. Prior authorization is becoming more important since many expensive treatments, especially those that may not be routine, are being challenged. A procedure that appears to be cosmetic may be a medical necessity in some cases.

It's very important to be sure of your coverage in situations where you might be referred to another physician, surgeon or hospital, i.e., you go to the emergency room or you're in the hospital and a consultant or surgeon is called in for an opinion or for carrying on your care. Your insurance may have covered you for your physician or for the hospital stay, but the consultants might not be covered. You should ask in advance so that you don't get surprised with big bills that aren't covered.

Medicare has phone numbers and web sites available for questions, as do some hospitals. Many companies that sell Medicare suppliers also offer assistance through local meetings or via the phone. You should have the name of your company with its phone number and the number of its contact people with you at all times, especially when you travel. Normally you have a card with this information plus the number of your policy and the name of the person the physician must contact for prior authorization, proof of current coverage, and any other questions that might come up. Before you get any medical care through a physician, hospital, outpatient facility, etc., you will be asked for this information. In many situations, if you do not have this information with you, you may be asked for a payment in advance and a guarantee that you will pay everything else directly.

If you have Medicare you need your Medicare card. Medicare-Part A covers hospital bills. For physician visits, you require supplemental insurance (Medicare-Part B). In general, Medicare pays for 80 percent of your costs and your supplemental insurance (or you) pays for the rest of the bill. You choose from a number of different plans, which are offered by many suppliers. Since deductibles, office co-payments and choice of physicians or hospitals can vary, make sure that you understand what's covered and if you're limited to certain providers or hospitals. With increased coverage, your costs go up.

There are many Medicare Health Plans (like HMOs, PPOs, Medicaid plans, etc.) that are approved by Medicare and run by private companies. Each often offers extra and/or different services, but may limit your access to care—meaning that you can only go to certain physicians or institutions, depending upon the policy.

To make it more confusing, there are also many pharmaceutical plans.

You should be informed as to what's covered on your policy. Many policies, including Medicare, limit your care to certain physicians and hospitals. There may be special expertise at one hospital or physician's practice, but the company will not pay for your visits to that physician or hospital.

Can you go to a specialist, i.e., an orthopedist or ophthalmologist, etc., on your own or must you get a referral from your primary care physician? Can you go to any physician or hospital that you desire? It's not uncommon to read about someone who has a disease for which care and treatment is extremely expensive, but find out that the insurance company has decided not to pay for them—or even discontinue payments during a costly treatment regimen. Often, the policies that offer the most benefits restrict your access to care, or have other regulations making it less convenient, but may be less expensive. Many policies offered by employers leave many gaps in the coverage.

The above comments are especially important if you travel since many Medicare, or private Medicare or private insurance policies, limit you to a certain local panel of physicians and hospitals. When traveling outside of your area, especially overseas, only a small part of your bill, or none of it, may be covered, leaving you responsible for the balance.

What are the rules in case you go to an emergency room or urgent care facility? Some companies will not cover some emergency room visits if they feel that you could have gone to a physician's office. This could be very costly to you. What services aren't covered? You may find out that you need care or exams that aren't covered in your policy. You should find out these answers early on since you might want to switch to another company, especially if you have a chronic or very expensive type of condition. It might be desirable to switch to Medicare, changing policies in the case of pre-existing condition.

If you go to a physician who recommends certain procedures that might not be covered (i.e., cosmetic surgery), the physician must check with Medicare or the insurance company beforehand to see if the procedure will be covered. If the answer is "no," he or she must have you sign a form that you understand this and will pay for it yourself. This must be done prior to doing the procedure. If it isn't done, the physician usually cannot charge you for the procedure. Be sure that you understand what's covered.

If you have coverage through an employer and are eligible for Medicare you might find that it is more desirable than what your employer offers. Medicare is amazing insurance, depending upon the plan, and is often less expensive and more inclusive than many private policies. This may change at any time.

Does your policy cover medications or do you have to buy a separate policy for medication coverage? If so, are you limited to generic medications or limited to where they must be purchased? Generic medications bought at a pharmacy outside of your plan may be less expensive than the medications allowed by your plan.

Can you still use your local pharmacy if desired? With many drug plans being offered, it's very difficult to make a decision. Research into the various plans is especially important if you're on special or high-priced medications that might be covered by one plan, but not by another. For medication coverage there are many different plans for drug coverage. If you're using expensive medications, find out if your drug plan will cover your medications.

If Medicare covers you, you may go to the following site for information: *www.Medicare.gov*. The following information describes some of the plans and is taken directly from the Medicare web site:

Original Medicare: This fee-for-service plan covers many health care services. You can go to any doctor or supplier that's enrolled and is accepting new Medicare patients, or to any hospital or other facility.

Medicare Health Plans (like HMOs and PPOs): These plans are approved by Medicare and run by private companies. When you join one of these plans, you're still in Medicare. Some of these plans require referrals to see specialists. They provide all of your Part A (hospital) and Part B (medical) coverage. They generally offer extra benefits, and many include prescription drug coverage. These plans often have networks, which mean you may have to see doctors who belong to the plan or go to certain hospitals to get covered services. In many cases, your costs for services can be lower than in

Original Medicare, but it's important to check with the plan because the costs for services will vary.

Medicare Prescription Drug Plans: These plans add prescription drug coverage to Original Medicare, some Medicare Cost Plans, some Medicare Private Fee-for-Service Plans, and Medicare Medical Savings Account Plans.

Medigap (Medicare Supplement Insurance Policies: These policies help pay some of the health care costs that Original Medicare doesn't cover. If you're in Original Medicare, you could get a Medigap policy to help cover the extra health care costs.

The amount of your coverage is also dependent on whether you have coverage under Medicare Part A, Medicare Part B, or both. Medicare Part A typically pays for your in-patient hospital expenses and Medicare-Part B typically covers your out-patient health care expenses.

A benefit is a health care service or supply that's paid for in part or in full by Medicare. Note: If you belong to a Medicare Advantage (formerly Medicare + Choice) plan, it must cover at least the same benefits covered under Medicare Part A and Part B. However, your costs may be different, and you may have extra benefits, like coverage for prescription drugs or extra days in the hospital. You should contact your Medicare Advantage plan administrator for specific coverage information for the plan in which you're enrolled. If you're interested in seeing what Medicare Advantage and Medigap plans are available in your area, please visit the Medicare Options Compare section of our website including doctor fees.

The following topics are among those discussed on the official Medicare site:

- Medicare premiums and co-insurance rates for the current year.
- Medicare prescription drug coverage—view an online demonstration on how to use the Prescription Drug Plan Finder.
- Medicare prescription drug plans—current plan data.
- Medicare health plans—current plan data.
- Formulary finder—current plan data.
- Lower your costs during the coverage gap.
- Learn more about plans in your area.

What is the future of Medicare in relation to your needs? There are many unanswered questions. The answers will evolve, but it doesn't appear as if there will be significant changes for most people in the near future. In summary, Medicare may be quite complicated and it's important to get the best coverage for you. Going to the official sites mentioned above may be helpful; otherwise you can call Medicare. I have found the site to be very helpful. You could also try calling your local hospital or AARP group for information. Be aware that your coverage and benefits may change in the future.

The Affordable Care Act: As in 1966 with the onset of Medicare, when there was much opposition to the "new" Medicare, we are seeing opposition to the Affordable Care Act. With the Affordable Care Act, when the details are worked out and when the system is able to function smoothly, it should be well accepted by patients and physicians. The availability of health insurance and care to many currently uninsured people will save many people from illness and death. Chronic diseases such as diabetes and high blood pressure will be treated with a sharp decrease in medical complications.

For the current Medicare patients, the ACA will probably have no effect on their insurance, their rates or their care. Many of the rumors, such as "death panels" (they do not and will not exist) are not true and should disappear as the ACA matures and becomes functional.

CHAPTER 11

Medical Costs—
How Do You Know?

What does medical care cost—in a hospital or in an office? Good question—and for a number of reasons, not an easy one to answer.

In general there's a cost for every procedure. However, this cost varies with each type of insurance—or no insurance.

- Private
- Medicare
- No insurance
- Medicaid

Since most patients have Medicare or some type of insurance, medical bills are often not examined. However, it's important to be interested and make sure that bills are correct—and if there's an error it should be corrected. It's extremely difficult to understand your statements from insurance companies or Medicare but you must make an effort. Unfortunately, although most physicians and providers are honest, there is too much fraud and the patient has a responsibility to report it if suspected. I would first call the physician, facility or hospital to get an explanation, which is usually satisfactory.

Medical offices and hospitals must have fee schedules for non-insurance patients. These are usually the highest fees and aren't paid by the insurance company. However, the patient without insurance, often on a limited income, is supposed to be charged these higher fees, even though it doesn't appear to be fair. These fees may be the basis for insurance payments, which might be a percentage of the non-insurance cost. This must be higher than what insurance pays since, if it's the real fee, the insurance carrier will automatically cut it, i.e., Medicare would only pay 80 percent of an allowed fee.

Many fees, especially hospital, are negotiated with insurance companies. This means that if a husband and wife have different employers, the fee paid to a physician or hospital for the same service might be quite different. Don't feel that the physician or hospital is trying to "gouge" the system. Medicare pays different prices to hospitals and physicians in different parts of the country, partially based on the area's cost-of-living. Private insurers will negotiate prices with each hospital in the area, resulting in different costs to the patient.

The "out-the-door" fee might be quite complicated since no one knows specifically what will be done when you walk into an office or hospital. Based on the initial history of your illness, many different tests might be required. You might have a simple cold which, because of what the physician finds in your history or preliminary exam, might end up being quite complicated, requiring extensive (and often expensive) tests. It's really not possible to know beforehand what the final fee might be because of the individuality of patients.

Negotiating with patients for fees is discouraged since physicians are supposed to charge what Medicare or the insurance company negotiates. If it's found that too many "discounts" are being given, the company may lower all payments to the physician, saying that the real fee is the discounted fee.

What can the patient do? There are a number of Internet sites that compare hospital costs and physician fees. However, do you want to go to a hospital or physician that charges lower costs if you feel the care is better at a higher cost physician or facility? Physicians and hospitals vary in their quality and the services they provide. Your goal is to get the best care possible. In general I do not believe in going to a facility, even one that is well-known, without a referral to a specific physician or clinic. I want to know who will have the responsibility for your care.

It still comes down to the fact that that patients try to choose the best physician for the current health care needs, and in turn go to the hospital where that physician has staff privileges. Medicine is still personalized—and rather than choose a facility, I always say choose the physician in whom you have confidence. There may be some variability in cost, but there's little to be done about it. If there's a true financial problem, many physicians and hospitals may lower costs to some degree. Ask—it never hurts to ask.

Often this is a moot point since most patients

have some type of insurance whereby they get complacent and totally ignore the bills. The insurance companies do not like physicians to charge lower fees for different patients. If you see that a physician or hospital bill is not correct, you have an obligation to explore this. I recommend that you first ask the physician or hospital about it. If you're not satisfied with the explanation, it might be necessary to contact the insurance company or Medicare.

You should be aware that the physician knows the least about most charges since we simply check a "code" for the procedure and the billing, etc., is then handled by someone in the office or hospital. And here's something you probably don't know: If a physician gets paid more than Medicare or the insurance company covers, we cannot keep the excess and must refund the difference to the insurance company or Medicare.

If the physician is not sure if Medicare or the insurance will pay for a procedure, he or she must have the patient sign a form that he or she will pay for the difference in payment or else, at least with Medicare, we cannot bill the patient for the excess amount. The physician may appeal a ruling before the procedure or afterwards if he or she felt it should have been covered. Afterwards, or in some situations, it's the patient who must ask Medicare or the insurance company to reconsider paying for a bill.

If the insurance company turns down payment before having a procedure, discuss this with your physician in order for you to decide how to proceed.

If you feel that you have been unfairly billed, then contact the physician, hospital or whatever facility did the billing to ask for an explanation. If you suspect fraud, you have a duty to contact the insurance company or Medicare. Billing and costs are often very complicated, especially with the hundreds of insurance companies with whom most of us will have contact.

CHAPTER 12

So You Think You're Paying Too Much?

There are a number of reasons why you think that a provider's bill for health services or supplies may be too high.

- The cost or fee may actually be too high.
- The cost may be too high for you.
- There may have been an error when the office was filling out the forms.
- The procedures may have been coded incorrectly.

The first thing you need to do before ever getting upset about a cost is to become more knowledgeable about the system—and if you think that health care professionals understand it completely, think again...but in any case, here are some basic concepts.

Most patients have insurance, which determines what the physician or hospital will be reimbursed. The amount is usually set by the insurance company with different companies often paying different amounts for the same service.

Office visits, exams, and procedures are in turn assigned a number, called a "code." Each code requires that certain care criteria must be met in order to cover the service provided—some codes paying the health care provider more and others codes paying less. And in order for us to get paid at all, physicians have to bill a certain—and, yes, unrealistic—amount but which in turn corresponds to a rate for patients without insurance.

Then the insurance company will pay a percentage of that "allowed" amount, i.e., Medicare will pay 80 percent of the allowed amount, regardless of what we're required to bill. This amount is somewhat arbitrary and chosen by Medicare or the insurance carrier.

In other words, insurance carriers apparently realized that costs could be lowered in the form of lower payments to patients by in fact lowering those fees to near the Medicare level. As noted earlier, physicians have to bill at inflated levels since Medicare or the company will pay a percentage of the fee charged, which in turn should be the fee which would be charged to someone who has no insurance, thereby significantly penalizing those who do not have insurance. Different carriers pay different amounts for the same code or procedure. Medicare limits the amount that might be charged.

The companies and Medicare routinely cut payments made to physicians and hospitals.

Thus, it's often difficult for physicians in certain fields to actually make a fair living. One way around this is to not accept Medicare and then otherwise charge higher fees than would be allowed by Medicare. In this situation, the physician advises you. You pay the bill and can still submit it to Medicare or your insurance company which will then reimburse you the fee that each usually pays.

Hospitals are having increasing financial difficulties because they are often reimbursed a relatively small fraction of what they bill each patient. At the same time, they must still provide free care to the indigent patient, especially in the emergency department. Hospitals in the same area may charge (or bill) wildly different amounts for the same procedure, although Medicare pays a standard lower fee.

As a patient, if you have financial difficulties, speak frankly to your physician or hospital. Physicians who take Medicare aren't supposed to waive co-pays or not otherwise charge patients unless patients sign a form saying payment cannot be made. When in need, ask your physician what can be done.

Be open with your physician or hospital. Many physicians will allow payments over time. In areas with teaching hospitals, there may be clinics that will accept you. However, these usually also have fees, but possibly at a lower amount.

If you find it difficult to pay for medications, ask your physician to see if he or the pharmaceutical company will provide drugs for nothing. This is not unusual. Unfortunately, physicians often now get few or no samples that in the past were so helpful to many patients in need. Also, in many communities, there are organizations that will provide medications.

If you're fortunate, you will have a Medicare or

insurance plan that pays everything without co-pays or deductibles. At the same time, it's important that you don't abuse this feature because it will cause increased costs for you and everyone else down the road.

Hospital bills are similar, but much higher. The bill often bears no relation to what the provider will receive from the insurance company or Medicare. Again, mention financial problems early. Some discounts may be possible. When you have extended and thus high hospital bills, the facility may be willing to give a discount. In this era of continuing cutbacks in reimbursement to health care providers and to hospitals by insurance companies and Medicare, it's becoming increasing difficult for physicians and other health facilities to handle the increased cost of rent, malpractice insurance, office staff and other areas of overhead.

Because of the enormous costs of most surgical procedures, a certain number of people are traveling overseas where orthopedic work, heart operations and cosmetic surgery are available at much lower costs than in the United States—but in some cases, also at a greater risk to the patient. It's especially important to evaluate any of these programs and/or providers carefully since many of them are excellent. However, your insurance may not reimburse you and many problems have occurred.

But the literal bottom line is that patients have a vital role in keeping some costs under control.

- If you have a full-pay or no co-pay plan, don't abuse the privilege.
- If you think a fee is out of line, or if you're charged for something that was not done, you must report it to Medicare or the insurance company. This is rare but does happen.
- If a planned procedure is not covered by Medicare, physicians must tell you in advance. You cannot be charged without signed permission from you in advance of the procedure.

In the end, the cost of providing health care is continually increasing, often putting it out of reach for many. There are no good, clear-cut answers, but we all need to help where we can.

Fraud and cheating are rare, but we must all be responsible and report it when it's suspected.

CHAPTER 13

The Reality And The Myth Of Prevention

It seems that many people who do not believe in prevention through "knowledge" are rationalizing that belief against a fear of finding out that they may have a disease. The truth is that most medical exams and screening exams reassure us that we're healthy, not sick. And since we can do something to treat many conditions, it's essential to have periodic medical and screening exams.

In ophthalmology, it's not unusual to examine people who are unaware of any vision problems and in turn diagnose diabetes, thyroid disease, glaucoma, cataracts, brain tumors, high blood pressure, etc., at a relatively early stage and thus allow intervention.

Glaucoma, if diagnosed early, often may be treated with preservation of vision for many years. Although we cannot prevent them, persons who have cataracts diagnosed in early stages can have blurred vision restored by simply changing glasses, thereby delaying surgery for a long time. Surgery is then carried out when vision cannot be improved with glasses

As well:

- High blood pressure, untreated, may lead to strokes or kidney, brain or eye damage. Early diagnosis, especially in African Americans, may be lifesaving.
- Unchecked dianbetes may cause similar problems. Early diagnosis and treatment may delay or prevent these seriously disabling or deadly complications.
- Death from colon cancer is almost completely preventable by regular physical exams and colonoscopy or its equivalent.
- Mammograms are used for early diagnosis of breast cancer.

It's hard to treat disease if it isn't diagnosed. We are making remarkable strides in treatment. Much research is being carried out in medicine that's directed to understanding the natural history of diseases. When that's understood, the next steps are directed to treatment and prevention.

The patient has a major role in this process. You must present yourself to a caring physician who's interested in not only treating your illness, but who's also concerned with preventative medicine. These two concepts are intertwined and should not be separated.

The patient should very much be the physician's partner in health care. As such, you must ask questions about both prevention and care. This will stimulate physicians to emphasize preventative medicine to a greater degree. Screening implies the use of a relatively simple test that will detect a certain amount of disease. By definition it will not be 100 percent.

The correct screening tests must be done. For example, screening for colon cancer is not adequate if one only depends upon stool samples for blood. Colonoscopy is required even though some cases may be picked up by the stool samples. In diabetes screening, urine tests aren't as effective as glucose tolerance or more sophisticated tests. No matter how sophisticated the tests, some cases will be missed. This is not a reason to avoid screening for disease.

Since there are tremendous numbers of tests that may be carried out for disease, the tests administered will depend upon your medical and family history and how these are interpreted by your physician. Although every medical exam could be considered a screening exam, your insurance also plays a role.

Medicare does not endorse routine physical exams on well people and, in general, does not cover screening exams unless there's a medical indication. This is changing. Insurance companies, in general, have policies to be followed for all testing. This will influence the decisions as to which screening exams are allowed. However, there are some diseases for which screening is covered by insurance—your physician will know which exams are covered.

Unfortunately many of these decisions are made on a cost-benefit (or risk) ratio. If a test is costly and will only pick up a small number of cases of a disease, it's often not reimbursed and not allowed by many insurance companies.

Therefore, discuss these possibilities with your physician since you may be willing to pay for certain screening exams yourself.

You cannot prevent many diseases. However, early detection may decrease the potential negative effects of certain diseases when diagnosed at an early stage and with the necessary treatments carried out.

Information on medical tests:
www.health.harvard.edu/fhg/diagnostics/

Home testing kits are available for many conditions. Ask your physician or pharmacist.

CHAPTER 14

What Was That Again?

It's been a universal joke for many years to poke fun at the handwriting of physicians. All that's necessary to understand the scope of the problem is to look at physician's office charts or almost any hospital chart and it's no longer funny. Medical charts are records of what has been done. Besides allowing for good patient care, it documents the exam, treatment, surgical procedures and what's told to patients. The legibility (and completeness) of writing will also serve as a significant protection for physicians in case of a claim.

Since most physicians use handwritten charts (this is changing), care should be taken to write or print legibly and in the necessary detail. An alternative is the use of scribes who are able to write legibly. The scribe is present during the exam and does all the writing the physician feels is necessary.

In addition, the scribe is present in order to get the patient in and out of the room, hand out the prescriptions, field any further questions, get instruments and generally help the physician see patients with more efficiency and accuracy. This of course means that that the physician is providing excellent care and taking the effort to provide the necessary detail for the patient's welfare and for the physician's protection.

With electronic medical records (EMR's), there is essentially no writing. However, the information must be typed into the computer and reviewed by the physician prior to "signing off" on the chart. They are quite expensive, but are subsidized by the government. Unfortunately they are not standardized, with many competing systems available. They also require intensive training of the physicians and office staff.

Whatever method is used, it's necessary to take a pertinent history of the present illness, take a past medical history, review medications and perform the necessary exam in the necessary detail with adequate documentation. Then the diagnosis must be clear, as well as the recommended testing and treatment. This would also apply to the surgical procedure and follow up.

When I look at legal charts of good physicians, it is frightening how difficult it's to understand the patient's problem and what was done due to illegible writing, and also incomplete information. If the matter becomes a legal one, this often results in a judgment against the physician since the written word (medical record) is the foundation upon which the court bases its final decision.

One complaint heard is that it takes too much time to document and to document legibly. As an attorney once told me physicians can either spend the time documenting legibly in the office or spend the time in court with him trying to explain what was done.

What's necessary to avoid these problems?

- A simple commitment to maintain legible, adequate records.
- Actually doing it on a regular basis.

Legible writing is something that we can all do if we feel it's important. Physicians should be objective and look carefully at all charts—and then should try to imagine an auditor or an attorney trying to read the charts.

Think about it.

CHAPTER 15

Talked With Any Patients Lately?

Obviously, this headline is a little facetious and a generality. However, it has a significant element of truth—and that's why I'm talking to my health care peers in this chapter.

Who cares?

- We (those of us involved with risk management) care.
- You care.
- And most importantly, the patient cares.

A major source of patient dissatisfaction—and with a certain percentage leading to malpractice actions against physicians—starts with us failing to talk, listen, and in a variety of other ways fail to communicate with patients. Note: I said "communicate," as opposed to "talk". . . and more importantly, communicate *with*, rather than talk *at*.

It's well known that physicians often do not allow patients to finish outlining a problem. Sometimes, and too often, the patient is interrupted after sixty seconds or less—and in a significant number of instances, if allowed to talk, the patient will allow the physician to make a diagnosis before even carrying out an exam.

A patient recently came to me for an eye exam. When paying and setting her return appointment, her husband (also a patient) was talking very loudly and critically about me. He asked her if I had done certain tests that would indicate a need for prisms in her glasses.

Hearing this, I suggested that she and her husband be brought back to an exam room so that I could discuss this with them and, hopefully, defuse a potentially serious problem. When I asked about his concerns, it turned out that he meant astigmatism, not prisms. He then learned that we obviously had checked for this. I explained the difference, what we had done, and asked if his questions were answered. He thanked me and left smiling.

Every exam is initially spent asking the patient about his or her problem and listening to the answer. At the end of the exam, I ask if there are any questions. If not, I tell the patient to feel free to call me at any time if questions arise, adding that, if I am not in, I will get back to him or her personally or via a staff member. Practically speaking, this "invitation to call me" has not been abused over the years.

If a patient cancels an appointment, the staff asks why and if there's been any problem. Either I, or a staff member, will call the patient back to discuss any concerns and ask if there are any questions. As in any business, if the patient's concerns are addressed promptly, roughly 90-plus percent will thank us and make a return appointment. Ignoring these simple concepts will allow patients who are unhappy to complain to his or her friends and acquaintances—or worse, end up on the wrong end of a legal action.

Most physicians are good physicians. Most

medico-legal claims against physicians are eventually dropped, but not without costing a significant amount of time, energy and money. Speak and listen to your patients and be available for questions and problems—this will surely decrease the chance of a malpractice action against you. Document these questions, discussions and answers and you will have a significant positive defense in the event an action is filed.

Be smart. Communicate.

CHAPTER 16

Management Of Lab Results —A Fly In Your Ointment

The management of laboratory and pathology test results may be a major cause of patient or malpractice complaints. Think of it—you're sick and worried that you might have a major health problem and the physician takes a biopsy or orders laboratory testing. You're waiting in a state of high anxiety, but don't hear from your physician for a prolonged period of time.

When you call the office, you're told that the results aren't back and that the doctor will call you when he returns from vacation in a week. You know that many results are available in a short period of time. The physician has three associates, but none will speak to you—and even if your doctor is in the receptionist will not connect you.

The above-mentioned scenarios are not unusual. Just listen to your friends at cocktail parties complaining about physician offices. No communication from a physician in general is also often a problem. When the patient calls, the results aren't available—either because the office can't find them or the specimen was lost or not sent out.

Any of the above may cause patients to become irate, especially if the test or biopsy results are bad and the patient feels that an earlier communication of results may have allowed a definitive operation or treatment to have been instituted, thereby saving the patient's life (from the patient's viewpoint) or, at the least, cut down on his or her pain and suffering. The patient is upset and complaining, only to be told by a friend that his or her doctor always gets back to him promptly.

How do we avoid these situations? Make sure your doctor knows that you want to know. Make sure he has your email address and/or web access. In our ever more technological world you may also want to consider having a printout of the lab results and, if applicable, a CD copy of X-rays or similar types of testing. The use of eletronic medical records makes this possible in most situations. You are handed a copy of your exam and lab test when you check out. Your doctor may offer this. Ask for the necessary information—and keep asking until you get satisfactory answers.

CHAPTER 17

Huh?

We take the ability to speak and communicate with others for granted. However, many people have difficulty with communication—and this may be dangerous to your health.

I'm not talking about a failure to understand this or that. I mean the more functional aspects of communication. Some examples are:

- People who are hard of hearing.
- People who are who cannot speak.

(list contiued on next page)

- People who speak a foreign language.
- People who have had a stroke or have neurological problems.
- An inability to speak after surgery.
- People with visual problems.

How might that affect you? Although you may have no difficulty communicating right now, you may develop a problem or you may have a spouse, relative or friend in this situation and you should be aware of what you can do.

Many hospitals have been aware of communication difficulties for a number of years and have developed systems to adapt. Whether it's in the emergency room, after surgery, or as a complication of a disease, the need for help may arise. Hospitals usually have large numbers of interpreters available for many languages, as well as sign language, lip readers and other means of communicating.

Be aware of what's happening. An individual may not respond because of the inability to understand directions or the inability to communicate concerns or simple questions. If you're involved with this person, take charge and ask for communication help.

Deafness is one example. When caring for these patients in the office, health care providers must provide an interpreter—at their own expense. This may cost the physician more than what's received for the care. Simply writing explanations or instructions or having a relative who does sign language is not sufficient if the patient wants an interpreter. There's an entire field of interpreters or medical communicators who are trained in medical terminology and who can explain medical questions or directions in a better way than those of us who do not use sign language.

Another example is that an individual may have an accident or stroke, followed by an inability to speak. This is very traumatic for the individual. Trained individuals who understand this medical problem can often communicate in a fashion that will reduce fear by a great degree. It may also allow health personnel to know that patient's problems and needs.

As friends or relatives, we should seek the help of someone to help improve this communication. It's often necessary for the friend or family member to bring up the need for interpreters at the hospital and about the need for an availability of communication assistance in specific situations.

In certain situations, the hospital must provide interpreters.

Sometimes it's the inability to speak English. The individual may be in pain or have a problem, but cannot communicate that need or can't provide the physician sufficient information to help in arriving at a diagnosis or to follow through on the recommended treatment. On occasion, I would have a family member come into the operating room to explain what's happening and calm down a patient who neither spoke nor understood English. It's quite traumatic to undergo anesthesia and surgery if you are not able to understand what's happening and what will happen afterward.

One area that comes up frequently is the individual who may not be able to speak due to a tracheotomy, or following a stroke. Think of the frustration involved with an intelligent person who's mentally alert but cannot ask for water, ask for a pain pill, or who cannot describe a problem that he or she is having. As family members or friends we must recognize this and ask for help. Sometimes, simply writing out the question or discussion and giving it to the patient will demonstrate that the patient can understand but can't talk or respond. It can also be a problem with physicians who don't speak English well and who don't understand the nuances that might be essential in making an accurate diagnosis.

In general, and in order to improve communication with all patients, physicians should supplement clear verbal instructions with written instructions as to what's wrong with a patient and how to use medications. The physician or a staff member should ask the patient if he or she understands the instructions. This should be confirmed by asking the patient to repeat the instructions—and repetition should continue until it's clear the patient understands.

In the hospital situation, recognize a problem that may not have been addressed by the staff. Don't be afraid to speak up and ask for an interpreter or someone who may assist in making things clearer to the patient or otherwise enable the patient to communicate. Be aware of possible communication problems among sick people and be pro-active in getting the necessary assistance.

CHAPTER 18

If You Don't Ask You Won't Know

You enter a physician's office, a hospital, or a testing center looking for a solution to your problem. You either:

- leave confused;

- don't understand the reason for the testing, medication or suggested procedure;

- or may not use the medications because of cost, not understanding the need, or perhaps not understanding the use process itself.

For some reason many people are afraid to ask doctors questions. Instead, many walk away confused, agreeing to procedures they don't understand, possibly resulting in poor health care. I, and many of my physician friends, have seen how many questions we get from our friends—about issues relating to their care by other doctors! There's no good reason for you to walk out of a medical office or a hospital without your questions being answered to our satisfaction. This is good reason to have someone accompany you to the office.

Why does this happen? Often it's because the information is not offered by the physician, or the office or hospital personnel. There's no good excuse for this. However, the primary reason is often that the patient or the family does not ask questions. Sometimes I hear: "I don't want to take the doctor's time," or, "the doctor gets upset if I ask too many questions."

A patient's anxiety may interfere with his or her abilty to "hear" much of what is said, or understand what is explained.

As physicians, we have an obligation and duty to explain what we're doing, what tests we order, why they were ordered, why surgery or testing is indicated, the potential complications of procedures, and whatever is necessary to make the patient understand and follow through with the recommended treatment. Not doing this may result in confusion on the part of the patient, not adhering to the recommendations and, often, not going back to the physician.

Sometimes this can result in serious illness, blindness, disability or death—and many of these problems may have been avoided if the physician had taken time to insure that the patient understood his or her illness and the recommended treatment. I always try to be proactive and ask if there are any further questions, ending every exam with directions for them to call the office if they don't understand anything, or if there are further questions.

Ask.

CHAPTER 19

Electronic Medical Records —A Salvation Or A Salve?

Electronic mdical records (EMR) have been pushed on the medical community almost as the salvation of medical practice and patient care. We were led to believe that information would be available immediately (and remotely) via EMR, and that we would become much more efficient because we would have more efficient offices. In large organizations such as the VA it's true that you can go into almost any VA facility and have all of your records available instantly. This is especially important for individuals who travel or spend time away from home—but it's not quite that simple.

There are some excellent systems but many aren't available to the average physician due to cost. To assist with this, the federal government has paid thousands of dollars to physicians who adopt an EMR system by a certain date. EMR permits the accumulation of much information that will always be available. Many physicians and hospitals like such a system, especially if it's been in place for a while—but there are some negatives.

There are many systems available with all degrees of sophistication. Most are costly and are often out of reach of many physicians. And with specialties such as dermatology, it's difficult to find a system that allows adequate drawing of skin problems.

There may be a long learning curve, which requires a significant reduction of patients, usually for a number of weeks, sometimes permanently. With this there's a significant loss of income, which may be permanent because of the reduction in the number of patients able to be seen. After adaptation, the EMR may add time to the exam because it takes time to enter the data—which also results in a significant decrease of income for a variable amount of time.

Although it was expected to allow better

communication between providers, this may not occur because of the large numbers of systems that often do not "talk" to each other. Even large hospitals may have several computer systems that aren't able to communicate with each other. Each allows gathering together much information quickly that should be readily available to another office, hospital or other health facility.

The major complaint that I hear is the interference with patient contact and care. It's often necessary to watch the computer and not be able to observe the patient and interact with him or her. This may result in missed diagnoses since facial and other expressions may be very important in making a diagnosis. However, this is diminished greatly with time and experience, or by use of an assistant who will input the information as the exam progresses.

Another significant concern is the apparent increase in billing to Medicare and insurance companies for services. With paper records it was felt that physicians often under-coded or forgot to code many conditions and situations. EMR systems allow itemization of everything done in the office with essentially automatic billing. Many of these charges were missed before EMRs.

There's a fine line between billing for services and the extra billing which is possible with EMRs. It's estimated that the itemization and the efficiencies will allow additional charges of billions. This is being watched closely by Medicare as well as private insurance companies. This is especially advantageous for hospitals that come out way ahead in contrast to private offices that may actually lose income.

As with many computerized systems, there is a danger of information being stolen or altered.

Electronic medical records have many advantages, such as the ability to receive, analyze and transmit large amounts of information efficiently. This is balanced by the decreased interaction with patients and the potential for a marked increase in billing. Such records are now here to stay, however, and should improve with time and experience.

CHAPTER 20

There Are Potholes On The Road To Quality Care—Ask

Availability of quality medical care varies tremendously. In many ways, it's proportional to the number of physicians and hospitals. Care is definitely limited without a reasonable number of both. And, although most problems may be handled by a good primary care physician, the need for specialists and super-specialists is self-evident.

If you're in smaller remote areas, these specialists may not be available or accessible. With modern transportation, this is less of a problem than in the past, but the time needed to travel distances for care may be critical in an emergency, and it may be prohibitive for an ill individual to travel for diagnostic and treatment necessities. Larger metropolitan areas may have a wealth of expertise in physicians, hospitals, including specialists, and super-specialists.

CHAPTER 21

Unhappy With The Doc? What Do You Do?

The following is a true story: A frustrated employee came to me for advice. Her child had a fever and was obviously sick. When she called her pediatrician, she was told that they could make an appointment, but it would be in a month—otherwise she should take her to the emergency room.

Beside it not being a true emergency, it would be extremely expensive. She took her daughter to the ER where she was evaluated, given antibiotics and told to see her pediatrician in three to four days. Upon calling the office, she was again told that the earliest appointment would be in a month.

What should she do?

My initial reaction was to tell her to find another pediatrician who was interested in providing good care. Usually, when a medical office accepts you as a patient, it means that the doctor will see you when you're ill.

Instead, I called the pediatrician and explained the situation. He was shocked and said that he would follow up. He said that what had happened was totally contrary to his philosophy. After checking with his office, he personally called the mother to have her bring the child in for the necessary follow-up.

As physicians, or as any other executive in business, we set policy and are responsible for staff following this policy. Especially in medical offices, physicians often enter the office through a side or back door and rarely, if ever, see what's happening in the reception area where patients are waiting. Doctors also do not see how staff interacts with patients and have no idea of how staff relates to patients on the phone.

How can doctors become aware of what's happening?

- Visiting the reception area during the day to see how people are being handled would be a good place to start.
- Looking to see if the day's appointments are actually on schedule.
- Listening to how the staff handles phone calls.
- Talking with patients and following up on anything that remotely sounds as if there might be a problem in the office.

It's fairly clear that the true story noted above does not appear to happen very often. But what can you do if it does?

When you have a problem with the office, speak to the office administrator or manager. If you do not get satisfaction, speak to the physician directly on your next appointment or before. You can also write a letter, marked personal—and I believe that the physician deserves this common courtesy.

CHAPTER 22

Still Unhappy? More Thoughts

Most physicians enjoy medical practice and want everything to run as smoothly as possible. However, many physicians want little—if anything at all—to do with administration and assume that staff is handling things appropriately. As with the physician in the last chapter, it's necessary to let him or her know if that isn't true.

Although there are some physicians who will deny there's a basis for your unhappiness, or in general shows not much interest in any problems —most will welcome your comments. The key is to present those comments in a non-confrontational, non-threatening way. In sum, try to talk *with* your physician, not *at* your physician—and if you're not satisfied with the answer(s), there's nothing wrong with leaving the practice.

If you decide to leave, first find another office that will accept you as a patient and make an appointment. Then contact your original physician well in advance to request that your medical records be either forwarded to the new physician, or are given to you to take with you on the first appointment. It's also nice to let him or her know the problems that you had with the office.

Although the records are in the physician's office, you have a right to receive the records yourself or to have the records sent elsewhere. Usually the state medical board will set standards for transfer of records with a fee that might be charged (usually a per page fee)—and some physicians will do this at no cost to you.

Recognize that, as physicians, we're there to help you and care for you. This involves seeing you when necessary or making provision for someone to see you in our absence. Any time that you go to a new physician you should ask for the office routine, i.e., how long does it take to get a routine appointment, or when you have a problem, how long does it take during regular office hours or after office hours?

However, if you have had a good experience with a physician and are satisfied with the care received but an unpleasant office situation arises, think first and discuss it with the office staff and/or the physician. Give the situation a chance to be rectified rather than go through the time and aggravation of taking your care to another medical provider.

CHAPTER 23

Medicine For All—
Telemedicine

A major problem in our medical system is lack of access to care and lack of access to physicians and specialists in many areas of the country. There are many communities with few or no physicians or specialists and many areas with no nearby, accessible hospitals. As physician assistants and nurse practitioners expand their roles, they will probably fill in in underserved areas.

As well, no physician has total knowledge and there are many situations in which an opinion or a consultation with another physician would be helpful. A partial approach to these situations is the field of telemedicine—accessing remote individuals, hospitals or medical centers for care that's not available locally. This is carried out through Internet access and may involve consultants from around the world.

As robotic surgery improves, it's conceivable that it might allow individuals in these areas to have surgery carried out remotely.

For many years, radiologists and neurosurgeons have been evaluating X-rays from home after hours. This has expanded to remote monitoring of X-rays by specialists twenty-four hours a day, often by radiologists overseas or by American radiologists. This gives access to super-specialists, not otherwise available, either in the hospital or off hours.

Computers and digital imaging have pushed us forward. Radiologists monitor certain neurosurgical procedures. When the radiologist is not available, this monitoring may be remotely available with the consultant speaking to personnel in the operating room via the phone, allowing critical surgery to go forward immediately, rather than doing it tomorrow or sending the patient out of town.

In the meantime patients in nursing homes or confined to home may have blood pressure, cardiac monitoring or other programs requiring continual evaluation followed remotely. Machines are now available to collect this information, as well as video for actually observing the patient wherever located. This allows almost instantaneous diagnosis of serious problems or a change in condition and may avoid the high cost of ambulances to take a patient in for evaluation.

It's well known that diabetic patients require yearly eye exams. Many primary care physicians now have special cameras and take pictures of the back of the eyes (the fundus). These are forwarded to an ophthalmologist, who may be thousands of miles away, for evaluation and diagnosis—thereby preventing much blindness.

It's also becoming more common for physicians to maintain contact with patients via the computer. It may be for making appointments, asking questions, or following patents with problems such as heart or blood pressure concerns, as well as many other disease conditions.

CHAPTER 24

Medicine For All— Telemedicine's Future

For neurological problems, it's often necessary to see a specialist. However, there's a severe shortage of some specialists, especially when a patient arrives in the emergency room after midnight with an unusual type of stroke or other neurological diagnostic problem. There are now techniques available whereby the emergency room physician examines the patient with a neurologist watching the exam on a television or computer monitor, giving directions and advice leading to a correct diagnosis and treatment.

Among the most valuable diagnoses is that of stroke; the immediate use of medications such as tPA (tissue plasminogen activator) a clot-busting drug can be lifesaving. This drug must be given early in the development of stroke and cannot wait for a referral to a neurologist the next day or days later. Due to many potential problems, it should only be used in certain circumstances and expert neurological advice is essential. Telemedicine allows the transmission of this advice.

This two-way video is also helpful in many other specialties. We now have companies that employ physicians twenty-four hours a day to perform telemetry that eliminates the problems for physicians not being available after hours or on weekends. Physicians in other countries may work during the day in providing care to countries that may be in night-time zones. This also cuts down on the fatigue factor, where some physicians may not be totally alert at 3 A.M. when called upon for advice. Telemedicine is also now coming into the average person's home wherein physicians are monitoring patients there, cutting down on sometimes difficult and expensive visits to the office or hospital.

Remote medicine has been experimented with

for over fifty years and is finally coming into its own. As time goes on, it should become more available and should save many lives at a significant saving to the patient and the insurance companies. At this time, however, many insurance companies will not pay for its use and most physicians and hospitals aren't geared up to use it. Contemplated future Medicare decreases may force the issue.

With the improvements in robotic surgery, it's conceivable that surgeons will be able to operate remotely, thereby making it possible for individuals living far from physicians and specialists to get surgical procedures that would have been unavailable previously.

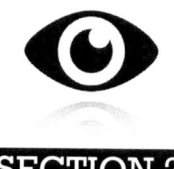

SECTION 2

More Than A Glance

CHAPTER 25

But It's Just Routine—Right?

In general, the practice of medicine is more exciting and more gratifying than ever before. The increased longevity and improved lifestyle of patients is proof that we are making diagnoses and successfully treating conditions that were never possible to treat in the past. With microscopes, gene therapy, DNA discoveries, use of stem cells, the ability to grow new limbs, etc., it's exciting to wake up almost every day to new advances.

An article in the *Wall Street Journal* (October 17, 2012) questioned the "value of medical checkups" (because they) "don't affect rates of death and disease." Eye diseases apparently weren't evaluated—and while most physicians in most general exams will perform some screening of patients for vision or eye problems, it's essential and sometimes lifesaving for some of the conditions discussed below to be diagnosed as early as possible—thus making routine eye exams essential.

At birth, premature newborns are examined (screened) for retinal damage for cataracts, tumors such as retinoblastomas, eyes crossing or turning out, and high degrees of near-sightedness or far-sightedness. In the pre-school age group, the same conditions may be discovered, as well as "lazy eye." There's always a debate as to the age of the first "official" eye exam. My feeling is that all children should have a complete eye exam at three to five years of age.

Although the yield of disease is relatively small, exams may pick up lifesaving or vision-saving conditions. When children have vision problems there may be significant difficulties in school. It's amazing to discover that a young boy can't see the school blackboard—but because he's yet to learn an adult point of reference, doesn't realize it.

The need for glasses may in fact develop

very slowly so that patients may have very poor vision and not realize it. These people are used to squinting, often developing headaches and not realizing the cause. It's not unusual for a patient to be unaware of serious vision problems until discovered on a routine exam. I have had adult patients with blindness in one eye that was never noticed by the individual until he or she had a problem with the good eye or simply had an exam for glasses.

Diabetes and high blood pressure are conditions that are often diagnosed on a routine eye exam—even though the patient may have seen a primary physician recently for a diabetic exam. These conditions might be quite advanced and detection may be lifesaving. Even when the patient is being followed by his or her physician, an eye exam may be the first evidence of poorly controlled conditions. Brain tumors, thyroid conditions or strokes may also be detected on a routine eye exam and before the patient is aware of them.

When patients have any of these conditions, eye exams are required at certain intervals to see if they are under control and if specialized eye treatments are indicated. Many eye conditions may cause a serious decrease in vision with the patient being unaware of the decrease that comes on so slowly that the patient adapts to it.

The two main conditions are cataracts and glaucoma. Cataracts may be easily treated with surgery, which usually restores vision. Unfortunately if glaucoma has been present for a long time, it may not be possible to restore any lost vision. Diagnosing these diseases must be done as early as possible. Early cataracts may have vision "restored" with a simple change of glasses. With early glaucoma, treatment with drops or laser may bring the pressure under control and preserve future vision.

Although certain medical exams may not be thought to be valuable in prolonging life, early diagnoses of eye conditions may not only preserve vision, but may also be lifesaving. Over the age of forty to forty-five years, routine eye exams are indicated every one to two years. With diseases (eye or systemic), testing may be needed more often. Preventive medicine is a major aim of ophthalmology and is very productive in terms of detecting disease.

CHAPTER 26

Whose Health Is It Anyway?

Are you coming to a medical office or hospital for health care?

Coulda' fooled me . . .

For whatever reason, it's often not clear why you're coming to a medical office for care when your actions show that you really aren't interested in your health, i.e.: negative vibes are given to health care providers:

- When you don't take medications.
- Don't keep appointments.
- Or otherwise ignore the advice your health care provider offers.

Patients often are very negative with health care providers (probably also with others in life). Yes, there are legitimate complaints: impolite staff, undue waiting, etc. However, impoliteness serves no purpose and usually makes the situation worse. And if there's a problem, notify the practice administrator or the physician directly. Occasionally, there's not a "fit" between you and a physician or a medical office—but if the care provider doesn't respond to reasonable requests, you certainly have a reason and a right to seek care elsewhere.

Be that as it may, and depending upon which study you read, about 40 percent of patients:

- Do not use medications correctly.
- Many in fact never get prescriptions filled.

Overall, it seems strange to go to a physician for care and not to follow through with the recommendations, i.e., the most obvious example is the prevalence of obesity. Patients may have:

- Cardiac problems.
- Diabetes.
- Or a whole range of diseases that obesity makes worse.

In spite of this (recognizing that it often is not able to be controlled), the obesity epidemic continues. No different with smoking, which is an addiction that must be treated as such. It's very discouraging to have a patient with major breathing problems come into the office with a package of cigarettes in his or her pocket, or to read about a patient on oxygen therapy who dies in a fire caused by the cigarette he or she lit while breathing the oxygen.

Smoking not only damages the lungs, but also may make diabetes or the eye disease of macular degeneration worse. It's well known that diabetics should have an eye exam annually in order to detect eye changes at a treatable stage. Recent evidence indicates that about a third of all diabetics have some eye damage. The only hope of keeping it from progressing is to have the patients come in for eye evaluations. Despite this being emphasized by the primary care physician, insurance companies and ophthalmologists like myself, many patients do not keep appointments and wait until blindness is already well underway (often too late) to return for ophthalmological evaluations.

Patients with chronic eye diseases such as glaucoma usually are seen every three to four months, often using two to three different drops every day. For whatever reason some patients stop using drops and don't return for several years, often with blindness (usually in one eye) as the result. I've never heard a rational explanation for this. Obesity and smoking are real problems that interfere with many medical and eye conditions. And with smoking, it's counterproductive to seek medical care when the obesity counteracts the recommended medical care.

It should be self-evident from what you have read, that you should:

- Listen to the recommendations of the physician.
- Ask for explanations of anything you don't understand.
- Write down complicated instructions.
- Use medications as directed and return for follow-up appointments as recommended.

Likewise, it's especially important today that you mention any financial problems that might interfere with your care. Physicians and hospitals are sometimes able to reduce or write off fees and often can make arrangements for you to get medications at a discount or at no cost, if necessary.

Communication is the key. Ask and listen. Listen and ask. You're a partner in your care. The physician wants to care for you, but you must do your part. And while a physician is not obligated to care for you, most physicians are interested, caring, and want you to get better and live longer.

At the same time, it sometimes comes down to what I mentioned earlier—the lack of "fit" between patient and care provider. When this happens the physician must give you sufficient notice to find a new physician and will forward a copy of your records. Sometimes personalities simply don't mesh; this should be recognized on both sides.

CHAPTER 27

Eye Problems And The Specialists

A number of eye questions will be discussed in this chapter. There are three primary groups involved in eye care: ophthalmologists, optometrists and opticians. More complete definitions follow.

Ophthalmologists (MD's) are medical doctors who have completed college, medical school and a residency in ophthalmology. They are licensed to diagnose and treat eyes and eye diseases, as well as to perform surgery (conventional and laser).

Optometrists (OD's) have gone to college and optometry school and are licensed to practice optometry. State licensing boards vary in what they are allowed to do. They examine eyes and treat eye conditions to varying degrees. Some states allow them to perform minor eye and laser surgery, and to use certain medications for treatment of eye diseases.

Opticians fill prescriptions, for glasses, that were written by an ophthalmologist or optometrists. In some states they also fit contact lenses.

The formal descriptions of ophthalmologists, optometrists, opticians and ocularists, as written by the American Academy of Ophthalmology and the American Optometric Association follow:

Physician

A person who has received the degree of doctor of medicine (M.D.) or doctor of osteopathy (D.O.) following completion of a prescribed course of study in medicine and surgery at an accredited school of medicine or osteopathy

Note: The definition of physician is provided here because federal law is sometimes used to include other health professions "for the purposes of reimbursement." This definition does not change the basic, generally accepted specific profession definitions that follow:

Ophthalmologist

A physician (doctor of medicine or doctor of osteopathy) who specializes in the refractive, medical, and surgical care of the eyes and visual system and in the prevention of eye disease and injury. The ophthalmologist has completed four or more years of college premedical education; four or more years of medical school; and four or more years of residency, including at least three years of residency in ophthalmology.

The ophthalmologist is a specialist who is qualified by lengthy medical education, training, and experience to diagnose, treat, and manage all eye and visual system problems and is licensed by a state regulatory board to practice medicine and surgery.

The ophthalmologist is the medically trained specialist who can deliver total eye care: primary, secondary, and tertiary care services (i.e., vision services, spectacle and contact lens prescriptions, eye examinations, medical eye care, and surgical eye care), diagnose general diseases of the body, and treat ocular manifestations of systemic diseases.

Optometrist

A health service provider who is involved primarily with refractive problems. Optometrists are specifically educated and trained by an accredited optometry college in a four-year course, but they do not attend medical school. They are state licensed to examine the eyes, determine the presence of refractive problems, correct refractive problems with glasses or contact lenses, and to detect and manage limited ophthalmic medical eye disease.

Optometrists work in private optometric practices, ophthalmology practices, multidisciplinary medical practices, hospitals, teaching institutions, research positions, community health centers and the ophthalmic industry. Optometrists can also build successful careers in the military, public health or government service.

There is a need for optometrists in all types of practice, particularly in the areas of pediatric and gerontological optometry. Practice opportunities exist throughout the United States with a particular need in rural areas.

Optometrists are required to complete a four-year post-graduate degree program to earn their doctor of optometry (O.D.) titles. The four-year program includes classroom and clinical training in geometric, physical, physiological and ophthalmic optics, ocular anatomy, ocular disease, ocular cytology, ocular pharmacology, neuroanatomy and neurophysiology of the vision system, color, form, space, movement and vision perception, design and modification of the visual environment, and vision performance and vision screening.

Optician

A professional, who makes, verifies, delivers, and fits lenses, frames, and other specially fabricated optical devices and/or contact lenses according to prescription for the intended wearer. The optician's functions include prescription analysis and interpretation; determination of the lens forms best suited to the wearer's needs; preparation and delivery of work orders for the grinding of lenses and the fabrication of eye wear; verification of the finished optical products; and adjustment, replacement, repair, and reproduction of previously prepared lenses, frames, and other specially fabricated optical devices.

Ocularist

A professional who designs, makes, and fits artificial eyes. And the following from the American Optometric Association:

As primary eye care providers, doctors of optometry examine, diagnose, treat and manage diseases and disorders of the visual system, the eyes and associated structures as well as diagnose related systemic conditions.

Optometrists examine the internal and external structure of the eyes to diagnose eye diseases like glaucoma, cataracts and retinal disorders; systemic diseases like hypertension and diabetes; and vision conditions like nearsightedness, farsightedness, astigmatism and presbyopia. They also determine the patient's ability to focus and coordinate the eyes, to judge depth and to see color accurately.

They prescribe eyeglasses and contact lenses, low vision aids, vision therapy and medications to treat eye diseases as well as perform certain surgical procedures.

CHAPTER 28

Can My Child's Crossed Eyes Be Outgrown?

Children rarely outgrow true crossed eyes (strabismus)—but there are things that your ophthalmologist can suggest. This condition should not be ignored. It should be evaluated promptly and adequately as soon as it's noticed.

A child with crossed eyes or eyes that aren't straight should be evaluated to rule out the presence of a serious eye disease that might be the reason for the eyes not being straight. This exam involves looking at the eye, evaluating the pupils and how the eye moves and instilling drops that will enable the determination of whether the baby is near- or far-sighted, or has astigmatism. It's essential to make sure that there are no other diseases, such as tumors, diabetes or others as the basis for the problem.

In addition, the drops make it possible to rule out the presence of diseases such as cataracts, glaucoma, tumors, scars and other conditions, many of which may be treated successfully if diagnosed early enough. The muscles are evaluated to determine which muscles aren't functioning correctly.

Crossed eyes in a child who's quite far-sighted often may be treated by the correct glasses. If there's any degree of accompanying amblyopia ("lazy eye") it should be diagnosed early so that treatment, usually patching the good eye, may be instituted. This is often quite successful if instituted early.

There is a condition called pseudostrabisms, which is when the eyes appear to be crossed due to a wide bridge of the nose. This is not true crossing of the eyes.

Another common eye muscle condition is exotropia—one eye turns out. Occasionally, glasses can keep the eyes straight, or the condition rarely can be improved with eye exercises.

If treatments (glasses, drops, exercises) of any eye muscle conditions aren't successful, eye muscle surgery might be indicated. For the horizontal muscles (when the eye turns in or out) this surgery is relatively routine for most ophthalmic surgeons. When the other (vertical and torsional) muscles are involved it's usually necessary to see a pediatric ophthalmologist who deals with these conditions more often.

CHAPTER 29

Can Near-Sightedness Progression Be Stopped?

My ten-year old is near-sighted:

- How might I stop this from progressing?
- Is this too young for contact lenses?
- If he gets contacts, will his near-sightedness be slowed?

Contact lenses may be fit at any age, usually being prescribed for medical, not cosmetic reasons. In an infant, a parent would have to insert and remove the lenses. They are especially effective after cataract surgery in an infant or small child, as well as when the child has lazy eye or a very strong prescription.

There is a feeling that prolonged reading and doing near tasks may make nearsightedness progress more quickly.

Various methods have been tried to slow the progression of near-sightedness, none of which have had consistent results. The amount of near-sightedness may be determined at any age. When very young, atropine drops have been used with mixed results. This is usually prescribed for daily use and cause blurring for near vision

As a child gets older, the main reason for wearing contact lenses is primarily for cosmetics and clearer vision than is attained with glasses. There's also improved clarity of vision in many cases, especially with strong prescriptions. Children usually start pressuring parents for contact lenses between ten and fourteen years of age, but contacts can be used at a younger age if the child is well-motivated and is dependable enough to follow instructions for proper wearing and care.

Although contact lenses may not slow or halt the progression of near-sightedness, that impression may occur because, since the lenses sit on the eye, small progressions of near-sightedness are less noticeable than in the individual wearing glasses. Also, since many individuals don't get contacts until older—and the eyes have stopped progressing naturally—contact lenses are mistakenly given credit for this. Clinically, the early teens appear to be the best time for contacts from the standpoint of patient adjustment and success.

There's a field of contact lens fitting called "orthokeratology." The results are still not in, but many optometrists and some ophthalmologists feel strongly that the special or specially designed lenses slow down near-sighted progression. This may involve wearing lenses over night to cause a change (temporary flattening of the cornea) in the cornea in an effort to reduce near-sightedness—often allowing the individual to see without glasses or contacts during the day. It does not appear to be a permanent improvement, but it is appreciated by many people.

CHAPTER 30

Glasses, Glasses—
The Differences Are Many

Glasses have two aspects, lenses and frames, and you want glasses that not only look good but also provide good vision and safety. There are many ways to purchase glasses:

- From a licensed optician.
- In the eye doctor's office.
- In a store or a retail chain.
- Via the Internet.

You should ask your ophthalmologist or optometrist for advice as to where to go for the glasses—and wherever you go, check prices and guarantees of satisfaction in advance. There are several potential aspects of problems. Glasses may be made incorrectly, may be poor quality, may be measured incorrectly, may be the wrong prescription or might not provide clear vision with either or both eyes.

When you need glasses there are a number of things that you should know. The first and most important thing to know is why you need glasses—and there are five primary reasons:

- Near-sightedness—can't see things clearly at a distance.
- Far-sightedness—can't see things clearly when close up.
- Astigmatism—an inability of the cornea to properly focus.
- Presbyopia—the need for bifocals as we get older (usually after forty-plus years of age)
- For protection—industrial, sports or general eye protection.

Except for the protective aspect, they are basically conditions where the shape of the eye is different, causing difficulty seeing—and glasses correct the way the misshapen eye sees.

And just to be clear, the reasons just noted above aren't diseases. These are instead vision issues caused by eyes that are misshapen or aging. (However, it's fair to note that in extreme degrees of near-sightedness, far-sightedness or astigmatism, these abnormalities may be responsible for eye damage or vision problems requiring special care or surgery).

When younger, there's more focusing power, enabling far-sighted people to see without glasses. As you get older, the eye loses its focusing power and glasses are then necessary to compensate for this so that you can perform near vision tasks. Over the age of forty to forty five, the lens loses its elasticity and focusing for near gets difficult— this is called presbyopia and is compensated for by the use of bifocals. Bifocals may also be used effectively to treat children whose eyes cross.

Glasses come in different forms. Single vision lenses, bifocal or multifocal, and lenses to correct the astigmatism are as follows:

- Single-vision lenses allow the correction of the distant or near vision.
- Bifocal lenses have a top part for distance and a lower segment for near, meaning

that distances between far away and up close will be blurring.
- Trifocal lenses allow correction of distant, near and intermediate vision.
- Astigmatism correction may be incorporated in any of the above lenses.
- Progressive lenses allow seamless transition between distance and near, allowing clear vision at all distances.

To avoid the in between blurring most patients are usually happiest with "progressive lenses" whereby all distances are clearly visible. These lenses come in a great variety of qualities with some providing better vision than others. Your optician can advise you as to the quality.

For most patients, these are the easiest lenses to use. In contrast to bifocals or trifocals, with progressive lenses there's no abrupt line in changing the distance at which you're looking, giving you a seamless range of vision at all distances. Progressive lenses are especially helpful for computer use or for individuals such as plumbers, carpenters and others who may work at intermediate distances.

In most cases where patients are unhappy with

multifocal lenses, I find that the lenses are either of poor quality or are measured (fit) incorrectly. Accurate measurement of the eyes and the frames is essential.

Then we also have glasses for the sun or for those who are sensitive to light. These may be sunglasses, Polaroid lenses or photochromic lenses (clear lenses which change color when exposed to sunlight). Polaroid lenses are excellent for those involved with water activities since you can see into the water for some distance, and glare is also significantly reduced.

When getting any of these, you should ask specifically if the lenses you're considering also provide protection from ultraviolet rays. The goal is to get as close to 100 percent UV protection as possible. Clear lenses usually do not provide any significant protection. The amount of UV protection varies with different lens materials—ask your optician for the details of the amount of UV protection and what might be best for you—and be especially careful with over-the-counter glasses.

There doesn't seem to be great differences with color, so get what you like since some people have preferences for certain color. Some colors, such as yellow, may enhance contrast making it easier to see a tennis or golf ball. Size of lenses is usually an individual matter. If the lens is too small, it may be difficult to find the correct area through which to look. Besides protecting the eyes, larger lenses will also protect the sensitive skin of the eyelids against sun exposure. Be careful when driving with sunglasses since there may be a problem if you have to enter a tunnel or if the sun goes down. Also, you may have a problem seeing in the house or in movies, but it will do no harm to your eyes.

Glasses may also be used for reasons other than simply seeing:

- Far-sighted individuals with crossed eyes, may respond to glasses by the eyes straightening, thereby avoiding surgery (especially in children as young as several months).
- "Lazy eye" (amblyopia) may be occasionally treated with glasses—with or without patching the good eye.
- People who are very near-sighted, far-sighted or with major degrees of astigmatism, may be legally blind without glasses and thus require glasses for daily functioning.

- Some individuals who are unusually sensitive to light (e.g., albinos) may require very dark special glasses to simply go outside.
- Some glasses have little "crutches" built into the frame for individuals with drooping eyelids, i.e., after Bell's palsy.
- Occasionally, an individual will have a disfigured eye or eyelids and want an opaque lens to cover this up.
- Lastly, essentially all glasses today should be made of plastic or polycarbonate plastic to provide protection in case of an injury. Anyone who works around construction, plays golf, tennis, contact sports, or engages in missile activities such as shooting or target practice should wear protective polycarbonate lenses with side-shields. Make sure that they meet industrial standards.

If you're going to wear glasses for industry, tennis, racquetball, home shop work, sports, etc., the lenses should be of industrial strength polycarbonate plastic inserted in industrial safety frames. For sports, frames with polycarbonate plastic are recommended. Sports frames have improved to the point whereby they may often be worn all of the time. Industrial and special occupational situations, i.e., welding or sports, may require special lenses and frames. Side shields are indicted in certain conditions. Ask your optician for advice.

Purchasing glasses through the Internet may create multiple problems, i.e., getting the correct measurements for frames, and more importantly, progressive, bifocal, trifocal and high prescription lenses must be measured carefully and inserted in frames that fit your face comfortably. The quality also must be evaluated.

Lastly, anyone with vision in only one eye or high degrees of near-sightedness may be more vulnerable to an accident. Such persons should consider safety lenses and frames full time, even if a prescription is not required. Accidents may happen at home or anyplace, and it does not pay to take chances. Ask your ophthalmologist, optometrist or optician for details about your glasses if you have questions.

CHAPTER 31

Don't Like Glasses? There Are Choices Beyond Contacts

In the '60's the idea of dispensing with glasses for younger people by operating on the front portion of the eye (the cornea) arose. Early on, many of those patients ended up losing much, if not all vision.

That operation is called "refractive surgery" and its use and improvement over the years has now brought us to the point where "lasik" and other refractive procedures can truly allow individuals to dispense with a reliance on spectacles for distant vision. It's often the first choice as an alternative to spectacles—and many choose it simply to stop wearing the dreaded glasses. And while bifocal refractive surgery is not possible at this time, monovision (correcting one eye for distance and the other for near) is becoming more popular. Correcting presbyopia (bifocal vision) with refractive surgery is being explored. When one gets to the bifocal age, it's necessary to use glasses for reading—these may be single-vision reading, bifocal or progressive lenses.

Times have changed whereby many ophthalmologists are recommending refractive surgery as the procedure of choice for many people who are near-sighted or who have astigmatism or in some children with amblyopia (lazy eye). These abnormalities may be responsible for eye damage or vision problems requiring special care or surgery. In addition there are individuals who wear extremely thick glasses who undergo refractive surgery. This results in markedly improved vision whereby everything looks larger and clearer—often undergoing personality changes (positive) due to their new, improved appearance without thick glasses.

There are also those who cannot or do not want to wear glasses, i.e., entertainers, military personnel, lawyers, or individuals who are routinely exposed to cold temperatures that cause glasses to steam up when going inside.

Refractive surgery in the military has become accepted and often required. With well over 312,000 laser refractive surgical procedures performed in the military since 1993, refractive surgery has achieved great respect. In a study of US Navy pilots, 100 percent obtained 20/20 vision and 96 percent attained 20/16 vision within two weeks of surgery. There was a 100 percent satisfaction rate, and 75 percent had 20/12 vision.

In the past, glasses or contact lenses were potential problems in some situations—and most obviously when taking a dive in an airplane. If the pilot loses drops or breaks his or her glasses, the result may easily be death to all on board the plane, and perhaps to others on the ground. Many persons requiring "strong" glasses were thus disqualified from flying because of these potential dangers.

Refractive surgery has been widely praised by the U.S. military, i.e., if a soldier in combat loses or breaks his glasses, he may not be able to recognize where he is going or who's shooting—an enemy or a friend. If captured, a soldier's glasses often are removed to make the soldier more vulnerable. In addition, refractive surgery now means it's not necessary to have special adaptation made to helmets, gas masks, etc. so that glasses may be worn. Navy Seals and others who perform water and diving duties are also much more effective after refractive surgery. Refractive surgery removes the need for glasses—and since vision is markedly improved, pilots benefit from an improved general and night vision.

Besides simply allowing the removal of glasses, there's usually an improvement of vision with most individuals attaining better than 20/20 (so called "normal" vision), often 20/10, without glasses. This improved vision allows personnel to function better and see in situations where lives are at risk. In the military we have the unique opportunity to follow large groups of patients in a standard way in order to evaluate the safety and efficacy of procedures. This information is usually not available in private offices where the number of patients is much smaller and different physicians may vary procedures.

For most people, laser refractive surgery is primarily cosmetic. However, when people or family members ask about lasik or other refractive procedures, recognize that many people have markedly improved vision over what's obtained with glasses, which may in turn help them at work and life in general. In turn, we owe much to the military for its role in protecting our country—and also for its help in evaluating medical advances in a way not possible in the private sector.

CHAPTER 32

I'm Having Trouble With My Glasses Or Contacts. Why?

Not everyone who gets glasses or contact lenses is happy. There are potentially a number of reasons for this and it's necessary to go back through the process to look for a cause. First, take your glasses to the optician (the person who sells and fits glasses) to see if he is able to find a reason. It could be:

- The glasses may not be the correct prescription due to an error in writing down the numbers. This can be a mistake in the doctor's office, may be an error by the optician in writing the prescription for the

glasses to be made, poor responses by you during the exam. Or there also may be a change in the eyes or the prescription since you were examined—even though it might be only several days since your exam. It also may be due to a general medical problem such as diabetes that's not well-controlled.
- The eyes may not have been measured correctly, especially with progressive lenses.
- The glasses, although ordered correctly, might not have been made correctly.
- The lenses may have been put in the frame incorrectly and may be rotated, or at an angle.
- Poor quality lenses aren't rare. This is a special concern when glasses are ordered over the Internet.
- Or you may need special adjustments for your occupation or computer use.

When glasses are ordered there are several measurements, i.e., the distance between the two eyes for reading and for distance, the distances between the two pupils, the distance from the eye to the lens, the height of the bifocal (in lined lenses) being too high or too low and the compensation for the eyes turning in when looking down. Any of these, especially with progressive lenses, may cause difficulty seeing. The lenses must be prescribed for your needs, i.e., a person with long arms might want his or her reading distance further away than average.

Each lens has a front surface and a rear surface. Especially in stronger prescriptions, putting the prescription on the wrong surface (the opposite of what you had in your current glasses) can be very uncomfortable. Switching from a lined bifocal to a progressive no-line bifocal may disturb some people. With the progressive, no-line bifocals it's essential to measure them correctly and to be very careful to coordinate the near and distance prescriptions.

When people order lenses online, it's difficult to get the correct measurements, especially in stronger prescriptions. There are also differences in quality among lenses, especially the progressive no-line lenses. Some cause tremendous peripheral distortion (patients say it's like the room wavering) and have different qualities for near and intermediate (e.g. for the computer) vision. Since there's also a significant price difference, the optician may use lower quality, less expensive lenses that do not function as well as better lenses.

With contact lenses the prescription may not be correct. Also, the lenses may not fit on the eye correctly. There are many lenses and types of materials that do not necessarily work for all people and all prescriptions. The most common reasons for dissatisfaction are:

- The wrong prescription.
- The wrong lens.
- The wrong materials.
- Failure to diagnose an underlying medical condition, which might require special lenses.

If you need bifocal correction, fitting with a single vision distant contact lens will not keep you happy in many cases. It's easier to fit the patient for a single vision contact lens and have him or her wear glasses for reading, but bifocal (multifocal) lenses have always been my preference if possible.

It's often necessary to be fit with specialty astigmatism, bifocal contact lenses, monovision (one eye for distance and one for near) or distant lenses with reading glasses. Strangely, some people buy lenses over the Internet or at gas stations or stores without being examined by a professional. Note that many cases of blindness have been reported, especially with colored lenses bought around Halloween.

If there's a big difference between the old and the new glasses or contact lenses, it may take a while to adjust to the new prescription. Occasionally, if you're going back and forth between your new and old glasses you also may be unhappy because of the difference in prescription or the size of the lenses.

If the optician cannot find a reason for you being unhappy, return to the doctor (ophthalmologist or optometrist) who originally examined you to see if there's another reason for you not being happy with your vision. Personally, the most common situation that I find is poor measurement or inferior quality of progressive lenses. It may be necessary to repeat the exam, even though it may be only a short time from the original exam. Your unhappiness with your vision may not have anything to do with the way the glasses were made.

First we recheck the examination for the glasses to make sure that the prescription ordered was correct and that it was written correctly. This may be due to poor responses on your part or may be due to diabetes, or you may have developed a medical condition such as cataracts. If you didn't have cataracts, some can develop rapidly, and your situation can change rapidly. There may also be a number of other medical conditions that may develop in the short time after the original exam.

If you're not happy with your new glasses, have the optician check them. If nothing is found, return to your ophthalmologist or optometrist to find an answer. Don't wait for a long time in the hope that you will get used to them.

CHAPTER 33

How Often Should I Have My Glasses Changed?

There's no specific answer to this. Your eyes should be checked regularly, especially if you notice a change in your vision. Glasses should be changed as often as necessary to improve variations in vision, not at specific time intervals. For example, the vision of children or that of persons with cataracts may change every few months (or more often), thereby allowing a significant improvement of vision with a change of the glasses' prescription, whereas some people might see well with a pair of glasses for many years. In these situations, when visual blurring is noticed, the individual should have another exam.

A sudden decrease in vision, even a day after you getting your new glasses, may be an indication of diabetes or rapidly advancing cataracts. It's normal to assume that there's a problem with the glasses, but there may also be a problem with your eyes that has suddenly appeared. I don't believe in saying that "you will get used to it."

Most people go back to the optician to make sure that the glasses are correct; but if this doesn't solve the problem, you should return to your ophthalmologist or optometrist to check to see if there's a problem with the eyes and not the glasses, i.e., check the prescription and look for conditions such as rapidly advancing cataracts, diabetes or other eye diseases. On the other hand, it's still necessary to have your eyes examined as indicated by your ophthalmologist or optometrist.

Without any diseases or problems being noticed, children should have a complete exam prior to entering school, then probably every five to seven years afterwards, unless the child has complaints or is referred from school. Over the age of thrity-five years, eye exams should be carried out every two to three years unless otherwise indicated. Patients occasionally are able to use the same pair of glasses for ten to twenty years. This should not give false reassurance that the eyes are healthy—routine exams are still necessary.

CHAPTER 34

Taking Your Contacts On Vacation

Contact lens use requires special care on vacations. Two things might be lacking:

- Clean water.
- The availability of cleaning solutions.

Before you depart, make sure that you have an adequate supply of solutions and lenses—the latter in the event you lose or damage those on your eyes. It's especially important to also have a pair of glasses in case you lose your lenses or if you develop an infection.

Take an adequate supply of cleaning, disinfectant and wetting solutions since your brand may not be available away from home. Do not substitute solutions or use generics unless you have no choice. Only use the solutions recommended by your doctor, unless you check first.

If flying on your trip, carry solutions in a clear plastic bag through the gate inspection. If you have any questions about regulations, call your airline or go to the Transportation Security Administration (TSA) website before going to the airport. After clearance, place contact lenses and solutions in carry-on bags in order to have them available during your travel and to avoid the temperature and pressure changes in checked baggage compartments.

Regardless of location, cleanliness is the primary problem with contact lenses in general—and especially when traveling. There are contaminants in all water supplies, so traveling may introduce new contaminants that might not be tolerated by your eyes. This may lead to mild irritation or major infections. In warmer climates (including in the United States) you're exposed to molds and many other bacteria.

Campers must be especially careful and avoid

swimming in rivers, streams and lakes with their contact lenses since they often harbor potentially blinding organisms.

We also know that under the best conditions, 60 percent of contact lenses are worn beyond the expiration date, some 70 percent of lens cases are contaminated from overuse and 25 percent are never replaced. When you leave your home to travel these habits may become disastrous.

Beyond the water issue, be especially careful about putting any lenses or supplies on counters. Carry disposable hand cleaners (sanitizers) to not only wash your hands, but to clean the counters. If you use the water to wash your hands, use plenty of soap. Try to avoid water in planes, trains or buses. Usually it's not suitable for drinking or for use with contact lenses.

Water supplies outside of the United States vary tremendously. The city water supply or the hotel or apartment water supply may carry many new germs. This is especially true in Third World countries and when hiking anyplace. In the wilderness, rivers and streams may appear to be clear and pristine, but are, in fact, major sources of potentially blinding bacteria. In areas of concern, there are small portable water purification systems that could provide safe water for hand-washing. Lens cases should be cleaned and put in boiling water every week for disinfection.

Under no circumstances—repeat, no circumstances—should you ever put your lenses in your mouth to wet them—unless you want to gamble with losing your vision.

If you're going to a specific area for a period of time, ask for the names of a local ophthalmologist or optometrist in case you have a problem. And regardless of where you go in the world, it's best to call your contact lens fitter if you have a problem. Contact lenses are wonderful—but you must do your part to ensure your safe use of them.

CHAPTER 35

Botox Has More Uses Than Mere Vanity

Botox (botulinum toxin, type A) and Myobloc (type B) are dilute solutions of purified dilute botulinum toxin. Botulinum injections in medicine, particularly in ophthalmology, have been used since about 1989. The dilute solutions have proven to be safe and effective for relaxing (actually mildly paralyzing) muscles in certain conditions. Under controlled circumstances, usually with monitoring of the muscles by an electromyogram (EMG), the muscles that aren't working correctly are injected. This will then weaken the muscle for months to years.

In ophthalmology we have been using Botox for over fifteen years in the treatment of crossed eyes. It's non-surgical and may be very effective. However, the early enthusiasm of this treatment has waned since it does not last as long as some surgical techniques. At the same time, it may be very effective and last for years, thus avoiding a surgical procedure and its risks.

With its marked effect on relaxation of the eye muscles, its uses for cosmetic reasons soon followed. Botox relaxes muscles for a variable length of time. Cosmetic Botox is used most extensively today for relaxation of brow furrows. Several essentially painless injections successfully improve brow lines in 90 percent of cases, giving a more relaxed appearance. However, Botox is often only temporary, lasting just one to four months in these patients. Nonetheless, patients are often extremely happy with the results.

Back on the purely medical front, and with varying degrees of success, Botox has been used for:

- Facial tics
- Migraine or tension headaches
- Dystonias—involuntary twitching of a muscle group

- Blephaorspasm—involuntary blinking or closing of the eyes that may be disabling
- Torticollis—spasms of the neck
- Involuntary facial muscle contracts
- Spasms in the legs
- Back pain
- Migraine headaches

As with any procedure, risks may occur:

- Infections
- Bruising
- Numbness
- Headaches
- Droopy eyelids

Over-reaction (paralysis) of muscles can also happen, but is rare. Injections should be carried out under sterile technique in order to minimize the risk of infections.

A qualified physician should perform Botox treatment. This would include an evaluation of the patient to determine whether it's indicated and to estimate the potential effect. Whoever performs the injections should be qualified to treat any potential side effects—and not merely someone with a needle. The physicians who perform these injections most often would include ophthalmologists, plastic surgeons, neurologists and dermatologists, although many other fields are getting involved.

Usually these treatments are for cosmetic reasons. That point is made because insurance is likely to cover the cost only if a medical reason is involved, such as disabling blinking of the eyelids. In these cases, the physician will usually evaluate the patient, and then ask the insurance company or Medicare to find out if it's covered.

A relatively recent phenomenon is the "Botox party." This is a type of marketing whereby a number of people are invited to a discussion of Botox for cosmetic purposes. Those who are then interested will have injections performed "on the spot"—often for a discounted fee. Botox has been an important addition to treatment options for many people and should prove to be more valuable in the future.

CHAPTER 36

Contact Lenses—Also Not Merely For Vanity

Contact lenses are miraculous pieces of plastic that provide many solutions to address patient desires and problems. The lenses come in soft and rigid materials and are usually used for cosmetic purposes, to be used instead of spectacles, or for medical, therapeutic purposes. The lenses used for medical purposes are the same or similar to the ones for cosmetic purposes.

Contact lenses may be used to treat certain diseases or to provide vision when it's not obtainable with glasses. There are patients with abnormal corneas (the front, clear "window" of the eye) who cannot be corrected to good vision with glasses.

The most common medical conditions in which contact lenses are used are keratoconus and scarred corneas. In keratoconus, the cornea is abnormally curved and may progress to the point of poor vision with glasses. These patients, and those with scars from various diseases and infections, often may have a rigid (gas permeable) contact lens placed on the cornea. The contact lens will have a thin layer of fluid behind it which thereby neutralize the irregularities of the cornea, providing excellent vision, and allows the patient to avoid having an operation—often for a lifetime.

There are also diseases or infections that may cause the cornea to be irritated and very painful. This may occur after injuries or eye surgery. Placing a soft lens on the eye will often relieve the pain and avoid the need for surgery. New procedures and techniques may restore vision without the need for formal surgery—a corneal transplant.

A patient may have abnormal eyelids, which may be irritating the cornea and may cause a loss of vision due to corneal scarring. Placing a protective bandage soft lens over the cornea may protect the cornea and maintain its integrity.

After refractive or corneal surgery, a soft, disposable contact lens may be used to minimize discomfort that may occur in some procedures. When a person sustains a scratch on the cornea, he or she might have severe pain. A "bandage" soft lens may be inserted to minimize this type of pain. Some people feel that this may also promote healing. There are also contact lenses that "self-destruct" or dissolve in one to several days for similar purposes.

An exciting area is new research using contact lenses to deliver medication to the eye. The lens is impregnated with a medication that is released over a period of time, allowing the eye to receive a constant and consistent medication level.

There are patients who are born without an iris—the colored portion around the pupil that regulates the amount of light that enters the eye. In this condition, an individual may be so sensitive to sunlight that it's almost impossible to tolerate being outside during the day. A darkly tinted contact lens, or one that's painted to allow only a small amount of light to enter the eye, may allow the patient to tolerate daylight and lead a more normal life. Other patients may have a seriously disfigured eye from an injury or disease. A contact lens may be painted to match the normal eye to decrease self-consciousness.

Fashion tinting of contact lenses is achieving greater popularity, as a fad or for making a statement. After 9/11, it was possible to get soft contact lenses with an American flag painted on the surface. Lenses are also available with logos painted on the surface. Other patients want to change the color of their eyes. This is now possible with a number of different lenses—and you can have almost any color eyes that you desire.

These lenses become especially popular at Halloween when they may, for some reason, be purchased, without an eye exam, at stores or gas stations. However, this dangerous practice results in blindness in a number of patients every year. Lenses should be worn only after a professional examination to determine the proper fit and safety.

Prosthetic lenses are painted shells to be used when an eye must be removed due to injury or diseases, minimizing any disfigurement. Although debatable, special lenses may be used for individuals who have a color deficiency—an inability to recognize colors. In lazy eye, an opaque contact lens may be used instead of the usual eye patch in a young child. For children or adults where an intraocular lens cannot or hasn't been used, a contact lens may provide essentially normal vision.

Although we normally think of contact lenses as a substitute for glasses, there are clearly—no pun intended—many other uses.

CHAPTER 37

Diabetes And The Eye— Your Role

Diabetes is a condition that may affect many areas of the body:

- Kidneys
- Heart
- Blood vessels (causing blood pressure problems)
- Eyes
- Skin
- Feet

However, how it can affect the eye is often the most feared. Occasionally diabetes may be diagnosed by the ophthalmologist due to the sudden onset of temporary, reversible complications such as double vision or temporary severe blurring of vision.

Although there are other conditions that may also cause these problems, when patients call with these complaints the first question I usually ask is whether or not they have diabetes because diabetes is the most common cause. With the diagnosis and initiation of treatment to control the blood sugar, these problems usually disappear and resolve completely.

Once diagnosed, the patient must become a partner in his or her care and make efforts to minimize potential complications. This requires a conscious decision that's often not easy. Diabetes may cause other problems before it's diagnosed. For example, on a routine eye examination we may see diabetic changes in the blood vessels (diabetic retinopathy) of the eye a long time before diabetes can be or has been actually diagnosed by the usual blood tests. Cataracts and glaucoma may also occur and require treatment. Therefore it's essential for all persons to, periodically, have a routine eye examination that includes dilating the eye and looking at the back of the eye for problems.

Once diagnosed, most physicians and ophthalmologists recommend annual dilated eye exams, looking for blood vessel or other eye changes that might develop without being noticed by the patient. It's essential for the patient to become informed and to develop a self-care plan. You're now a partner with your physician. Although the physician can prescribe medicines, a new lifestyle is essential. It takes great commitment to follow the regimen of medications, diet, weight control, etc. Educate your family and friends so they may help you adhere to your regimen by not encouraging you to eat foods that may not be good for you.

Diet and exercise are amazingly effective in decreasing, and often reversing, the effects of diabetes. This is most dramatic when bariatric surgery is performed on obese patients, often resulting in elimination of the need for insulin and major improvements in the general health of patients. However, and unless the patient continues to monitor his or her weight, the diabetes may return. Unfortunately many people with diabetes suffer severe eye damage, which would often be diminished or avoided by good control of the diabetes.

Diet is probably the most important factor in controlling diabetes. It's well known that poor diet, being overweight and using nicotine are factors that may adversely affect diabetes and vision. Also, use of alcohol may cause a lowering of blood sugar and may interfere with good control.

Besides the annual eye exams, your primary physician must follow you annually or more often, as indicated. "Diabetic retinopathy" is often the most feared complication of diabetes. This is the involvement of the blood vessels in the retina at the back of the eye. New vessels in the retina may appear and result in damaging bleeding. If this occurs, laser treatment and injections of new medications may be of limited value in the restoring of vision and in stopping the progression. However, intensive research is improving the prognosis. Besides protecting the eyes, the above comments are also important in reference to protecting your, heart, skin and kidneys—all of which may be involved with diabetes.

In summary, diabetes may affect the eyes. In order to prevent or minimize problems, the patient must partner with the physician and take charge of his or her care and modify his or her life accordingly.

Some sources of additional information about diabetes are:

The National Eye Institute (NEI)
The NEI is part of the National Institutes of Health. To learn more about eye problems, write or call the NEI:
2020 Vision Place
Bethesda, MD 20892-3655
Phone: 301-496-5248
www.nei.nih.gov

For more information about taking care of diabetes, contact:

National Diabetes Information Clearinghouse
1 Information Way
Bethesda, MD 20892-3560
Phone: 1-800-860-8747
TTY: 1-866-569-1162
Fax: 703-738-4929
Email: ndic@info.niddk.nih.gov
www.diabetes.niddk.nih.gov

National Diabetes Education Program
1 Diabetes Way
Bethesda, MD 20814-9692
Phone: 1-888-693-NDEP (6337)
TTY: 1-866-569-1162
Fax: 703-738-4929
Email: ndep@mail.nih.gov
www.ndep.nih.gov

American Diabetes Association
1701 North Beauregard Street
Alexandria, VA 22311
Phone: 1-800-DIABETES (342-2383)
www.diabetes.org

Juvenile Diabetes Research Foundation International
120 Wall Street
New York, NY 10005-4001
Phone: 1-800-533-CURE (2873)
www.jdrf.org

CHAPTER 38

Most People Have Cataracts?

A cataract is a cloudiness of the lens of the eye and no surgery is required unless it gets dense enough to interfere with vision, or the health of the eye. Most people have cataracts. Fortunately, nine out of ten do not require surgery.

Persons who do have cataracts are normally followed for years before vision problems develop. However, a cataract may progress very rapidly (rarely, in days) to the point where the vision is sufficiently impaired. This could be mild to severe blurring of vision or severe disabling glare. It's not necessary to wait until you're blind to have surgery. Actually, due to the progress in cataract surgery, many people are electing to have surgery much sooner than in the past.

Cataracts may be a complication of trauma or many medical conditions; medications such as cortisone can also cause cataracts. When decided upon, almost all cataract surgery is done in an outpatient setting, either a hospital or an ambulatory facility. Usually one eye at a time is operated upon with the other eye having surgery within several weeks. Some ophthalmologists are performing cataract surgery on both eyes at the same time. This is not generally done out of fear that, if a rare infection occurs, it might damage or blind both eyes. Often the other eye may have good vision and may not require surgery for many years. Almost all surgery involves removing the cataract and replacing it with an intraocular lens.

What are the decisions that you must make? First, all decisions are based on communication with an ophthalmologist. You must decide upon the surgeon, and if you have an ophthalmologist, make sure that he or she performs cataract surgery since many do not do this. If he doesn't perform the surgery, ask for a recommendation. If you do not have an ophthalmologist or optometrist, you can get names from your primary care physician, local medical society or hospital—or perhaps from a friend. To some degree you may check him or her on the Internet to find out qualifications or potential problems.

Many insurance programs have lists of providers that you may use or have to use. If you go outside of this list, the company will often pay less and sometimes pay nothing at all. This also applies to the facility where the surgery will be performed. You must have this information before you undergo the surgery in order to prevent potentially expensive surprises.

Once you opt for surgery, you must decide when (or where) to have it done. Fortunately, complications rarely occur but usually the surgeon likes you to be in town for two to four weeks after surgery in case there are any post-operative problems. Unless your insurance requires the use of certain facilities, you may have a choice—and ophthalmologists often operate at several locations.

CHAPTER 39

On The Other Side Of The Scalpel

I am writing this several hours after my own cataract surgery. What was it like for an ophthalmologist to be the patient? The view from the other side of the scalpel is certainly different.

It started at 6 A.M. and upon arrival at the outpatient surgery center in Canton, Ohio, I encountered a model of efficiency and caring. Most of the time was spent answering questions and completing paperwork. After signing the necessary forms, I was taken to the pre-op area where I removed my shirt, donned a gown, got on a gurney, had an IV started, and saw my doctor—after which I was taken to the operating room with almost no waiting.

Flawless efficiency and a flawless team effort were obvious. After saying hello to everyone in the operating room, the next thing I remember was getting ready to walk out to go home. I had been given a small amount of medication in order to avoid any pain sensation. The only discomfort lasted about five seconds when the first drop was placed on my eye. The short-acting medications eliminated all pain. The painless procedure was over in less than half an hour. In retrospect, the major inconvenience was getting to the surgical center at 6 A.M. since I wanted to be the first patient of the day.

My wife drove me home and I took a short nap, after which life returned to normal. I stopped by my office to get some temporary glasses and went for a walk prior to starting this article. My vision in the operated eye is improving rapidly. Six hours later the vision in that eye is better than would be needed to pass a driver's test and I am able to read the newspaper with slight difficulty.

I chose a toric (astigmatism) single vision implant which would eliminate my astigmatism, but I still need a bifocal for near work. Insurance will not normally cover these special astigmatism and multifocal (bifocal) implants. I "cheated" and had a lens made up (for my glasses) for my operated eye beforehand—a bifocal with no prescription for distance so that I would not have the blurring that my old lens would incur. Although not covered by insurance, I would highly recommend this. Some people simply take out the old lens for their frame, but they then don't have the bifocal help. It's fairly easy to calculate this beforehand, recognizing that it may have to be changed later.

What a change from when I started in ophthalmology. Back then patients were kept in the hospital for a week, had very limited activity for three months and did not get final distorted vision glasses for two months (unless I fit them with a bifocal contact lens, which restored very normal vision quickly). The procedure entailed painful injections and a prolonged recovery period.

After six hours I was essentially back to normal activities (driving to be resumed in the morning since the minimal anesthesia prohibits driving for twenty-four hours). I still had some slight blurring of my right eye, but I was rapidly improving each hour. I would go out to dinner this evening, resume driving tomorrow and exercise and tennis next week.

After about eight hours, my vision returned to almost 20/20. The most noticeable change was that everything that was white was perfectly clear with the right eye and is now noticeably yellow with the left eye due to the cataract, which never appeared to bother me very much (It can sneak up on you). The vision improves during the day since there may be a slight fluid buildup in the cornea (front surface) of the eye that disappears over a number of hours, giving better vision later in the day.

My summary of day one: a painless operation with rapidly improving vision causing essentially no discomfort or inconvenience. The vision was quickly passing that of the better, un-operated eye that was not bothering me until I saw the improvement from the operation and could compare the two eyes. For a short period of time, I will be wearing a protective shield over my eye at night (in case I bump it by mistake). I will also use drops three to four times a day.

It's hard to see why people would hesitate to have this operation if it's indicated. I see too many people in my office who need cataract surgery but put it off because of fears of surgery. This is not to minimize or negate the real concerns of possible complications (glaucoma, retinal detachment, infection, etc). Cataract surgery is not always successful; complications can occur during and after surgery and must be carefully considered by the ophthalmologist and patient prior to doing surgery. Fortunately, the vast majority of patients are happy.

Day two was similar to the end of day one—back to normal activities, driving, etc., but still avoid major exertion, exercise, etc. I am able to ride my exercise bike, walk and do general exercises. It's nice to take it a little easier. In spite of the bright sun, I don't have to wear my sunglasses and vision continues to be excellent. Fortunately there's still no discomfort and my operated eye feels the same as the other eye The only difference is that there's a little sticking of the eyelids, getting better quickly, as I am up and I blink a little more often. Reading fine print is a little difficult, even with the glasses.

Day three and beyond—normal activities. The eyes may take a while to attain the final, best vision and glasses; each person is different. By day four the distant vision is 20/20 and reading the newspaper is relatively easy. Some ideas to make it a little easier:

If there's much sensitivity to bright lights, wear the sunglasses. Use common sense and follow your ophthalmologist's instructions. Some of us are more conservative than others. I will be resuming my exercise routine, but will avoid lifting weights over twenty-five pounds for a week or so. Otherwise, my activities were back to normal two days after surgery. I'm back seeing patients and resuming my ophthalmology practice obligations.

I suggest reading the newspaper on the computer since you can make the print as large as you wish—if you have any difficulty with the fine print of newspapers. In addition, the black and white format makes it easier to see than the actual newspaper where there's much less contrast. Near vision is a little fuzzy at first.

Return to normal activities as soon as you feel comfortable. At a minimum, if possible, take walks, which will make you feel better and more confident. Don't be discouraged if your vision is fuzzy, especially if you haven't changed the lens for the eye that had surgery. It's often good to have that lens of your current pre-operative glasses removed since it was prescribed for your vision before the surgery. If you have had a multifocal lens, it may take a while for you to adjust to the new vision. If you have a choice, I would suggest asking your ophthalmologist to "guess" at the post-operative vision and prescribe a lens for use the day of or after surgery—this will not be covered by any insurance.

As a patient and as an ophthalmologist, cataract removal has made amazing advances. Some of us remember the stories from before my entering ophthalmology. Patients were instructed to:

- Keep the head from moving.
- Refrain from bending over.
- Not lift anything over five to ten pounds for three months
- Expect two to three months of recuperative time before the vision stabilized when the final, extremely thick and unsightly glasses would be prescribed.

I'm pleased to note that none of this holds true today, and that cataract surgery has achieved an amazing level of rapid vision restoration.

However, it should only be undertaken when needed—basically when the cataracts interfere with your normal functioning. Just keep remembering that it's still an operation with all the potential risks that might occur with surgery. Rarely, problems may occur during the operation, or weeks to months to years later. My fondest hope, however, is for everyone to do as well as I did.

CHAPTER 40

Your Doctor Doesn't Have X-Ray Vision

Don't let poor vision sneak up on you. Cataracts, glaucoma and diabetes may be responsible for a painless loss of vision that may come on so gradually that you might not even realize that you can no longer see adequately. There are many conditions that might be detected during routine exams, and which may be at a state where vision might be restored or where visual loss may be halted. They may only be detected if you have periodic eye exams.

A cataract is a clouding of the lens of the eye. It's not unusual for the patient to have a gradual decrease of vision to the extent that he or she is legally blind and didn't notice the loss over time. Nine out of ten people with cataracts don't require surgery—they may have their vision improved with glasses. However, when glasses no longer provide clear enough vision and your daily functioning is compromised, removal of the cataract with implantation of an intraocular lens may restore essentially normal vision.

Cataract surgery is elective and is usually not necessary if the vision is good and the individual is getting along well. An exception to this might be where a patient is doing well, but has a condition at the back of the eye that must be monitored by the ophthalmologist and may not be clearly visible due to the cataract. Examples of this might be diabetes, glaucoma or macular degeneration.

Strangely, some people allow themselves to go blind from cataracts by failing to get a simple exam. It's understandable that these people are delighted after successful cataract surgery. Modern cataract surgery is carried out in an ambulatory center that might be in or associated with a hospital, an accredited free-standing facility in an ophthalmologist's office. Free-standing facilities may vary significantly in quality and care. All surgical facilities should be accredited as meeting the necessary standards.

No or minimal medication is used and the patient returns to essentially normal functioning and activities about an hour after surgery—a major advance over the old-fashioned days of sand-bags and poor vision for weeks to months. The surgery is quick (twenty to forty minutes, plus time for preparation for surgery). In essentially all cataract surgery, the cloudy cataract lens is replaced with a modern marvel—the intraocular lens. These implants may correct for distant vision, astigmatism or bifocal needs.

Diabetes may affect the eyes. The most important factors in preserving vision and reducing visual loss are annual (or more often as necessary) ophthalmologic exams, adequate control of blood sugar, weight control and exercise. During the eye exams, diabetic changes in the back of the eye may be detected and special photography (fluorescein angiography) may be carried out to determine if laser treatment is necessary. When indicated, laser treatment is highly effective in controlling visual loss.

Glaucoma includes a series of conditions in

which the pressure in the eye is high and can damage the nerve at the back of the eye, resulting in vision loss. It's often diagnosed on a "routine" exam. A sudden type of glaucoma, angle closure, results in severe headaches or pain in the eye with blurring or loss of vision, causing the patient to seek care. Note that African Americans often have no pain and may have serious damage before seeking help. The pain may be relieved with return of vision with use of the laser, usually in the office or in a hospital facility.

On examination, the ophthalmologist usually sees the predisposition to this type of glaucoma. This is explained to the patient so that he or she does not ignore the symptoms of an acute attack. Often, a laser iridotomy (opening in the iris, the colored portion of the eye) is made with a laser in the office in order to prevent future problems.

The more common chronic open angle glaucoma is often picked up during the "routine" eye exam. It's more common if members of the family have this type of glaucoma. Diagnosis by the ophthalmologist is made by looking at the nerve at the back of the eye in conjunction with measuring the pressure and side, peripheral vision). Treatment involves the use of drops, and/or laser or other surgery. This type of glaucoma may respond well if diagnosed early.

Modern ophthalmology is not only concerned with medical, laser and surgical treatment of diseases. We are dedicated to the principal that prevention is the most effective "treatment." It's not possible to prevent eye disease without regular visits to the ophthalmologist, especially when specific high-risk conditions, such as diabetes, cataracts and glaucoma, may exist or be in the family. Conditions such as tumors, high blood pressure and many more may also be found in a routine exam. Recognize that even with regular visits, diseases may occur which isn't always curable—but also that there are far more which can be dealt with successfully.

CHAPTER 41

The Second Opinion— Wait A Second!

Fortunately, most conditions for which we consult our physicians are relatively straightforward and can be handled by our personal physician. And many, if not most, conditions will resolve with little or no medical help. Lastly, there are many excellent, caring physicians in most communities.

The generally accepted notion is that everyone should have a primary physician who can be called in the event of a medical problem. This physician should be accessible and you should have confidence in him or her. However, when you start with a physician there should be some ground rules:

- When should you call him or her?
- What should you do if you have questions?
- Can you run the question by the office to see if you have to be seen, or is it always necessary to make an appointment and go to the office? This is especially important with complex or serious conditions that may occur. Sometimes a simple question may be answered on the phone.

However, there are rare times when you may want to exercise your right to get a second opinion. It may be for something that's being treated in the office or hospital, or it might relate to surgery or other complex or disturbing conditions.

Will your physician "allow" or object to this? This usually comes up in the course of treatment and is typically not discussed beforehand. Patients are often reluctant to ask for a second opinion, primarily because they don't want to "upset" their physicians. In fact, some physicians will object strongly or get upset. However as physicians, we don't "own" you, meaning that you can ask questions, seek another opinion, etc. Nonetheless, physicians are only human and may get hurt or upset if you question an opinion or recommended care.

In this new era of medical care, patients are often very knowledgeable and may find information about care that the physician doesn't have. Patients are also emotionally involved in the problem and for a number of reasons may not be happy about the progress or the treatment plans that are being proposed.

Communication with your physician is essential. Ask questions, but recognize that a certain number of physicians don't like to be questioned. In these situations, you must decide if this is the correct physician for you. If there's a concern, it's best to discuss it with your physician since he or she may not realize that questions appear to be discouraged. Also, many physicians prefer to finish doing all the diagnostic workup before getting involved in discussions since new test results may change everything dramatically. However, there are times when questions become necessary because of the complexity of a case or because of complications. This might be due to chronic pain, fatigue or any condition that cannot be diagnosed relatively quickly. The body is very complicated and may not respond clearly to the diagnostic routine or the treatment involved.

When you have concerns, it may be necessary to stop and review the situation. Speak to your physician to see if there are any unknown problems or concerns and if he or she is comfortable with how things are progressing. If you're not making any progress or if you have concerns as to what's happening, you might be interested in a second opinion. First, you should discuss this with your physician, mention your concerns and see if he agrees with you.

And then you should read the next chapter.

CHAPTER 42

Second Opinions— A Few Seconds More

Think you need a second opinion?

No matter what concerns you, you should discuss it with your physician. I have always tried to suggest the possibility of a second opinion before the patient brought it up. Usually the patient would refuse it, but there were situations when I insisted because a second opinion or a consultant might have treatments available that were not available to me. Sometimes it was important to reassure the patient about his or her visual problem.

It's relatively rare for the second opinion to offer new information, and it usually confirms what you already know. However, it's best to get your physician to make the referral and to "stay in the loop." This is because there are situations where the consulting physician may have information or treatments available that have not been available to your primary physician—and you would obviously like to know about these.

What are the negatives of second opinions?

Some might be confusing since the consultant may make recommendations that are significantly different than what has been recommended. At that point, you should discuss this with your original physician since the new opinion might not be correct for you. You must make a decision as to which opinion is the correct one.

Another negative is that the second physician is also not as familiar with your case, along with that, getting a second opinion may delay care needed for the condition involved. As well, a second opinion may be inconvenient and costly, and may not be covered by your insurance, especially if it's "out of network." In order to get the second opinion, there may be a significant delay in treatment. If it entails staying in the hospital longer, this cost may be passed on to you. Clarify this before seeking the opinion.

In summary, you're always entitled to a second opinion. This should be discussed with your physician and then evaluated with his or her assistance and input. Although it's relatively rare that the second opinion offers new information or treatment, it does occur occasionally.

CHAPTER 43

So What's An Advocate?

With hospital gowns being all the same it's hard to distinguish among patients. Other patients often may have the same last or first name or a similar name. It's not unusual for medical personnel to come in the hospital room and automatically assume that you're the correct patient. Your ID badge is supposed to be checked and your name asked. However, if the patient is confused, or if the person asking for this information does not have fluent English skills to discuss the medical condition or a medication, an answer is sometimes given automatically without really understanding the question.

Persons may come into the room to take the patient for testing, X-rays or surgery. It also might be to give medication, start or continue intravenous treatments, etc.—but do you know? Usually, but not always, the person offers an introduction. You can simply ask the person for a name and position in the hospital. If there's any concern, do not be afraid to ask for the nurse in charge to make sure that everything is correct.

A major problem may arise when the patient is very ill and may be lethargic or confused due to the medical condition or medications. In these situations it's good if a family member is able to stay with the patient. Some people pay for a nurse or other individual—an "advocate"—to stay with the patient, even to the extent of going to the operating room area with the patient. At the same time, it's absolutely imperative that anyone who's helping with the patient not interfere with hospital personnel.

It's essential that patients be informed as to what to expect in the hospital. Similar concerns are also valid in the physician's office. All personnel should introduce themselves and explain what they are doing. In the office situation, patients are often anxious and do not understand what's being said or what's being done. Because of this, it's usually a good idea for a family member or friend to accompany patients to the office, and take notes as to diagnoses, medicines and testing. The patient may be having reactions to medications or other problems that are not recognized by the hospital staff and not able to be verbalized by the patient.

And in the next chapter, it's even more critical that everyone knows who you are.

CHAPTER 44

What Hand Am I Holding Up, Doc?

We've all read the stories about a doctor amputating the wrong leg or otherwise operating on the wrong site. Early in my training I had the unfortunate (however fortunate for the patient) experience of notifying my professor that he was operating on the wrong eye. Fortunately for the patient and the doctor, it was the beginning of the operation and no damage was done. This experience remained with me, always making me take extra precautions to avoid the same mistake when I was doing surgery.

I once had someone tell me that her podiatrist

operated on her left foot when it should have been the right. Also, someone else told me that in the operating room the nurse insisted that his surgery was scheduled for his left leg when it should have been the right. Since the nurse could not be convinced, he got up from the operating room table and left the hospital. He then found another surgeon who would take better precautions to avoid a similar problem.

What can be done to prevent these needless situations? First, recognize that many people are involved in your surgery—you, the surgeon, the nurses, and all the ancillary personnel—and it begins with you. You must show interest in any procedure that involves you. Make sure that you understand what's to be done, what medications are to be used and don't be afraid to "check" by asking questions and volunteering information: "You know that my operation should be on my left hand?"

If the patient is not alert, a family member or friend must take charge to try to avoid this type of potential problem.

The wrong site surgery issue has been recognized nationally, and with the Joint Commission on Accreditation of Healthcare Organizations

(JCAHO) coming out with a protocol that's endorsed by over forty professional organizations. Unfortunately, it only applies to any hospitals, ambulatory care or office-based surgical facilities that are accredited by the JCAHO. If you're about to have surgery, you can ask if the facility has this accreditation or if it follows the required protocol. It basically involves continually checking and rechecking by everyone.

There are a number of common sense procedures to follow. Preferably, the surgeon should clearly mark the site on which surgery is to be performed. The surgeon should verify this mark with his or her initials. In ophthalmology we tell patients that they will be asked many times "which eye is to have surgery today?" It doesn't mean that we're not sure, but we just don't like to make mistakes. We also mark a big "X" above the eye that's to have surgery.

When in the operating room, the surgeon should have your chart and recheck everything, including the proposed site of surgery. A relatively new innovation is the "time-out" before beginning the operation. The patient's name is checked as well as the consent form, what type of surgery is about to be performed, and on what part of the body. This should be verified by the nurses, assistants, the surgeon and the patient if he or she is awake.

Recognize where errors may occur. When surgery is proposed to the patient, it should be clearly documented in the chart. However, when the surgery is scheduled, this involves someone calling from the doctor's office and someone on the other end of the line writing down the information. This is then placed upon a number of sheets, or in the computer, any one of which may be done incorrectly. Recently approved abbreviations have been recommended to avoid problems in interpreting the physician's handwriting or abbreviations. Occasionally the patient is anxious or confused about the surgery site and tells the staff that it should be on the other side of the body. This should be rechecked. If family members are present it may be necessary to involve them.

What should happen if the surgery is performed on the wrong site or the wrong operation is carried out? While this is extremely rare, it still occurs too frequently. However, most facilities have a protocol in place for handling these problems. This starts with the surgeon discussing the problem with the patient and the family, not only in respect to what has been done, but what's recommended to be done next.

More information on this topic may be found at: *www.jcaho.org* and *www.aao.org*.

CHAPTER 45

What Constitutes An Eye Emergency?

The major emergency requiring immediate care is a chemical injury, whereby something splashes in the eye. In this situation the eye should be irrigated or washed out as fast as possible with water. If there's no water, use almost any non-chemical solution.

Pour the water in the eye or actually place the head and eye under a faucet for several minutes. Don't waste time trying to figure out if the chemical is an acid or alkali. The worst are the alkalis that may not look so bad, but will often get worse as time passes. Fortunately, most substances that are splashed in the eye cause no permanent damage.

With fireworks injuries, cuts of the eye or lids, and other types of major trauma, avoid pressure on the eye. The patient should keep the eyes closed gently, following which the patient's physician should be called or the patient should be taken to the emergency room. No bandage is necessary since this might place undue pressure on the eye and potentially more damage.

If something blows into the eye, often it can be flushed out with water, or may be removed with a tissue if you know how to turn over the eyelid to look underneath. If it's on the clear cornea (front surface of the eye), it's often necessary to see your ophthalmologist or optometrist, or go to the emergency room if it cannot be flushed out.

An allergic reaction may cause marked swelling of the clear covering of the eye, appearing like a large bubble or blister on the eye surface. The eye may also get very red and the lids may become very swollen. Cool compresses may be very effective. If not, consult with your physician for medications.

Sudden pain with redness and blurred vision, as well as any sudden loss of vision, should be handled by calling your physician immediately or by going to the emergency room. Since many physicians, especially ophthalmologists, prefer to see the patient in the office situation where more equipment might be available, it's usually desirable to call your ophthalmologist or physician first for instructions prior to going to an emergency facility.

In addition, you should have an idea of what constitutes an emergency for other parts of the body, for example, breathing, heart, legs, etc.

CHAPTER 46

What Should I Look For In An Eye Exam?

An eye exam should inform you:

- Whether or not you need glasses.
- Determine the presence or absence of disease.
- Recommendation whether or not you need glasses, medication or any treatment.

The examination will vary from office to office but will include certain fundamentals. A history is taken to discover past injuries, illnesses, medications, allergies or anything else that might affect vision. Specific visual concerns and complaints are targeted and addressed. The vision is checked for near and distance with and without your glasses. Depending upon the office, various automated exams may be carried out by a technician prior to seeing the ophthalmologist or optometrist. The exam to determine the need for glasses, and the strength of the glasses is carried out. In addition the pressure may be checked and photographs of the inside of the eye may be taken.

Depending upon the office, all of the above may be performed by a technician before you see the ophthalmologist or optometrist, who will then carry out an en external exam to evaluate the eyelids, eye muscles, pupils and the conjunctiva (clear covering of the eyeball). The bio-microscope is then used to look at the clear window (cornea) of the eye, the colored portion (the iris), and the lens. This will pick up scars, inflammation and cataracts.

If not done before, the pressure is checked as a small part of the exam for glaucoma, usually under a blue light. Drops to dilate the pupils may also be given. Drops are usually used to make the pupil large for examination of the back of the eye the retina. At this time the nerve is examined for evidence of glaucoma or tumors. The blood vessels are checked to see if there are any harmful effects of diabetes, high blood pressure, kidney disease, circulation problems or a myriad of other conditions.

The above are the basics of an exam that will vary according to the findings in each part of the exam and the needs of the patient, i.e., contact lens exams will require different tests. On the other hand, when a patient is evaluated for a specific problem, only a portion of the above tests, or other tests, would be done.

CHAPTER 47

Aging And Your Eyes

As individuals age certain changes in the eye occur normally. And in our forties is when things generally begin to change, as follows:

- It becomes more difficult to focus the eye for near tasks, resulting in the need to wear bifocal glasses.
- Colors may become less intense and there may be a generally slight decrease in sharpness of vision, with a decrease in side (peripheral) vision.

- Most noticeable for most people is the need for more light, especially at night, causing driving to become more difficult. In addition, glare becomes more of a nuisance and situations in which contrasts of objects are decreased will impair visual functioning.

The above changes occur gradually and usually we adapt to them quite well with minimal disruption of any activities. However, in disease situations such as cataracts, macular degeneration, glaucoma, diabetic retinopathy, circulation problems, complications of surgery or unsuccessful eye surgery, or strokes or the above changes may become exaggerated and disabling. With cataracts, the visual disability may usually be removed with successful cataract surgery and intraocular lens implantation. In many other eye conditions medication, laser and surgical procedures may only stabilize or halt the visual loss, but will not usually return the vision to normal.

What can be done to help the patient who has poor vision and needs visual rehabilitation? First, a thorough eye evaluation must be carried out to be sure that there's no treatable or correctable eye disease. Then the extent of visual loss and how it interferes with the patient's functioning must be determined.

A careful refraction (exam for glasses) with some additional magnification will enable most people to perform everyday tasks such as writing checks and reading their mail.

It's important to find an ophthalmologist, optometrist or other facility for a low vision evaluation and recommendations. There are many devices available for a multitude of low vision problems.

For watching television, sporting events or looking for the number of a bus, special magnification telescope systems are often effective. If reading standard print is too much of an effort, most local libraries carry large print books, talking books, e-books and magazines. There are also crossword puzzles and many games in large print.

When high degrees of magnification with special lenses and optical systems are necessary, careful instruction is required to assure success in their use. Recent advances in television and reading magnification systems, with a decrease in their cost, enable many people with poor vision to continue their employment in the work force without interruption.

For people who work with computers, special large print software is miraculous. This enables use of the programs used by other better-sighted employees. For specific details on the above means of improving vision, more information should be requested of your ophthalmologist or optometrist. You may also find further information at the following sources:

American Foundation For The Blind (AFB)
15 West 16th Street
New York, NY 10011
Phone: (212) 502-7600

National Library Service For The Blind And Physically Handicapped
Library of Congress, Washington, DC 20542
(800) 424-8567
www.loc.gov/nls/

National Center For Vision And Aging
The Lighthouse
111 East 59th Street
New York, NY 10022
Phone: (800) 334-5497

Bureau Of Services For The Visually Impaired
400 Campus View Boulevard, Sw3
Columbus, OH 43234 4604
Phone: (614) 438-1255

The Council Of Citizens With Low Vision
Kalamazoo, MI
Phone: (616) 381-9566
www.cclvi.org

CHAPTER 48

Falling—And Not In Love

Everyone trips and occasionally falls. Is this serious? It certainly can be if you break a bone or sustain other major injuries. According to an article in the May 2004 issue of *Ophthalmology* falls are amazingly common as we grow older. According to the 1992 *Annual Review of Public Health:*

> Falls are a common cause of morbidity and mortality in the elderly. Approximately one third of older individuals fall each year, and seven percent of individuals older than

seventy-five years have an emergency room visit for a fall-related injury each year. Approximately six percent of urgent hospital admissions among older individuals are secondary to fall-related injuries.

Why do people fall? There may be many reasons. First, one may simply trip over something such as a curb. Renouned dietician Dr. Robert Atkins slipped on the ice and fell, sustaining a head injury that led to his death. A recent non-scientific poll in Canton, Ohio, revealed that about two thirds of people in Canton slip on the ice and fall at least once during the winter, whereas about 20 to 30 percent of people slip and fall two or three times during the winter—a good reason for being in a warm climate and avoiding the ice.

There are medical reasons why people fall. In the *Ophthalmology* article, the study found a significant increase of falling in elderly individuals who have vision problems. The study concluded:

> A change in vision over approximately a five-year period is an important risk factor for frequent falls. Thus, to decrease the risk

of frequent falls and fall-related injuries, older individuals should be referred to eye care providers not only when there's loss of (visual acuity), but also when the (visual acuity) can be improved with cataract surgery or correction of uncorrected refractive error, such as with new eyeglasses or contact lenses.

Vision problems accounted for a significant increase in hip fractures among women. The types of vision problems that occur and that might contribute to falling may be:

- Poor vision—difficulty seeing the chart clearly can cause a two to ten times increase in falling.
- Decreased side vision—as may occur in glaucoma or with strokes.
- A change of vision that may occur with cataracts or macular degeneration.

When older individuals fall, larger issues sometimes occur. Simply, bumping your head or any fragile bones can cause injury. This may be especially serious if the individual is taking anticoagulants. With aging, bones become more brittle and coordination difficulties make it more difficult to avoid damage by breaking the fall.

Putting the arm out to break the fall often results in breaking the arm. Twisting, when falling, may cause hip fractures or tears of muscles or ligaments. Hitting the head may result in brain hemorrhages and other brain damage that may result in death. In fitness centers and hospitals, there may be exercise programs for older individuals to improve balance and review proper falling skills so that injuries might be avoided. Besides treating the fall itself, as physicians we try to determine why the person fell:

- Is it simple tripping, or was the fall a result of passing out or loss of consciousness as may occur with a stroke or tumor?
- Is there a neurological problem? Often, even if there's no obvious damage, we must still seek a cause for the fall.

Obviously we try to determine what type of damage has occurred and make a decision as to whether or not the patient may be discharged from the emergency room or admitted to the hospital.

How can we avoid falling?

- Be careful. Look where you're walking. Try to look for uneven sidewalks, obstacles in the way, sunken living rooms, missing bricks in a sidewalk, etc.
- If you have difficulty seeing, whether at night or during the day, look more carefully and avoid areas where you might not be able to see obstacles.
- At home, place a contrasting edge (a different color of paint or an edge) on stairways or steps, especially when going outside.
- If you have several steps or a sunken living room, have a railing.
- In colder climates think twice about walking outside if there's snow or ice, which might cause you to fall.

Many individuals are unsteady, whether due to muscle problems, neurological issues, or other balance problems. A major safety factor is the use of a cane. Too many people look at a cane in a negative manner and place themselves at major risk of falling by trying to avoid using it. Don't be afraid to use a cane when necessary because it may save your life. If you do fall, be evaluated as necessary to see if there has been damage and if there's a curable cause as a reason for the fall.

P.S. Don't be afraid to use a cane. And if you must fall—fall in love.

CHAPTER 49

Having Trouble Driving At Night?

As I get older I notice more difficulty driving at night and reading? Why is this? From childhood on there are natural changes in the eyes that decrease our ability to see as well at night. For some people over the age of fifty this will cause enough of a problem that night driving may have to be avoided. And even for persons with 20/20 vision, it's not unusual to hear complaints about difficulty reading highway signs during the day, as well as at night.

Aging causes a decreased ability for the eye to function well in the presence of glare and also a decreased ability to rapidly change focusing on objects. The glare from the headlights of oncoming cars (especially if you have cataracts) may make it impossible to drive. This glare "intolerance" may apply to reading situations also. The eye also requires more contrast to see at night as well as for reading.

Another factor is the need for more light to see as well as in the past. Add this to the decreased contrast at night and it can be very difficult to drive after susnset. Contrast how a twenty-year-old zips easily around a dark neighborhood while an older person has difficulty finding the driveways.

Increased lighting may also be necessary for reading. With e-book machines, it's easy to increase the contrast or enlarge the print for more comfortable reading. You can also change to white letters on a black background, which may be helpful for many people. Often, all that's necessary is a change of glasses. Deterioration or other eye diseases may require more effort for you to read and will also contribute to eye fatigue. With macular involution or any other conditions of the eye, there's no harm in continuing to read or using magnifying glasses to read.

As for driving, there's no harm if you can meet the vision requirements. You may have to drive a little slower and more carefully. However, if you cannot meet vision requirements or if you do not feel comfortable driving, do not drive since this might endanger yourself and others. Many people limit driving to driving only near home. This is faulty reasoning since most accidents occur within twenty-five miles of home. If you have any doubts about your ability to drive, ask family members or friends as to your general safe driving ability—and consult with your eye specialist to see if you meet the vision requirements. Difficulties in reading should also be mentioned due to the many modalities available to assist you.

CHAPTER 50

You Want To Celebrate Having An Eye Injury?

It's a tragedy that many people—and especially children—will lose some or all vision during holidays or other celebrations. The American Academy of Ophthalmology's Eye Smart program says that certain precautions should be taken to protect children's eyes when choosing gifts:

- Select toys and gifts appropriate for a child's age and maturity level. Avoid toys with sharp protruding parts like pellet or paint guns, rifles and darts.
- If you're giving sports equipment, be sure

to include appropriate protective gear, such as helmets, facemasks or goggles. These gifts can reduce eye injuries by 90 percent.
- Christmas tree branches and needles can be hazardous to eyes, so be especially careful when untying or decorating your tree. The branches can quickly burst forward, injuring your eyes. Hang all glass ornaments out of a child's reach to avoid any potential harm.
- New Year's is often ushered in with fireworks. Attend professional fireworks displays—never allow children to play with with fireworks or sparklers, because there's no safe way to handle them.
- Even opening champagne can be dangerous. Be sure corks are pointed away when opening a bottle. Prevent the cork from popping off uncontrollably by covering it with a towel and slowly turning it with a slight upward pull. It's important to keep the bottle cold; sparkling wine should be chilled at least 45 degrees Fahrenheit before opening.

CHAPTER 51

What Is Vision Screening?

Screening exams, for any condition, is basically the use of a relatively easy technique or exam to pick up certain diseases. It's not foolproof and will not pick up all people with these diseases.

Blood tests screen for glaucoma; spine measurements screen for scoliosis; mammograms check for breast cancer; etc. For eyes, we screen for poor vision in children, glaucoma, diabetes, macular degeneration, etc.

As for school eye exams, they are screening exams given by nurses and/or volunteers and aren't complete, professional exams. The vision is checked, using an eye chart, usually by trained volunteers or nurses. Nonetheless, such exams are extremely worthwhile, being responsible for discovering many cases of amblyopia ("lazy eye"), as well as many cases of poor vision.

By definition it should be understood that school screening is not a complete, professional, diagnostic eye examination and that failure of this exam does not necessarily mean your child requires glasses. However, screenings can help in vision education and picking up many eye conditions at a stage when treatment is possible.

Screening for glaucoma entails checking the eye pressure with or without looking at the back of the eye.

Macular degeneration progression is often detected by looking at a grid of small squares and noticing if there are blank areas in the vision.

Although a certain amount of disease is detected, requiring referral for definitive diagnosis of disease, a major reason for health screening is education.

For more information on vision and eye health, visit: *www.geteyesmart.org*.

CHAPTER 52

What Determines The Color Of Eyes?

Although heredity is a major determinant of the color of your eyes, the actual color depends on the amount or concentration of pigment in the colored portion of the eye called the iris.

All colors are determined by the brown pigment called melanin. If there's very little melanin, the eye is grey or blue. This color is often related to the amount of pigment elsewhere in the body. The determination of color depends upon genetics. Each parent passes on two pairs of genes. The eye has multiple factors in the determination of the final color, with the OCA2 gene being most influential. Since other genes may also contribute to the eye color, there may be a number of variations of color.

In other words, an individual with a fair complexion (due to less melanin in the skin) often has blue eyes and light hair. These individuals often have a decreased tolerance to the sun and may have more sensation with contact lenses. Such persons may burn more easily and have more discomfort in bright sunlight, thus requiring skin creams and ultraviolet absorbing sunglasses in order to enjoy the outdoors on bright days. With darker skin, more melanin is present causing the eyes to be brown. Less pigment tends towards lighter eyes. Albinos have essentially no pigment in the eyes and therefore no protection. This may make it impossible to go outside during the day due to the resultant light sensitivity.

CHAPTER 53

Lasers Are More Than Science Fiction

The laser (Light Amplification by Stimulated Emission) is basically a concentrated beam of energy, created from gases such as argon, krypton, CO2 and neodymium:yitrium. This energy can be used to cause reactions in the eye by heat (argon and krypton absorption of the laser energy by the pigment of the retina or blood vessels) to in turn cause a heat-type reaction which will act like spot welding to seal a retinal hole in the case of a flat retinal detachment, or to seal off areas in the treatment of diabetic damage to the eye. The laser is also used to treat inflammation and bleeding in certain disease conditions such as histoplasmosis and wet macular degeneration.

The Nd:YAG laser causes bursts of energy, which are used to cut tissue such as part of the lens of the eye to prepare for certain types of cataract operations and to destroy residual membranes or scar tissue that may form after cataract implant surgery.

In the field of glaucoma, lasers are used to create openings in the iris (iridotomies) for the treatment of angle closure glaucoma or to lower the pressure of the eye in open angle glaucoma by making small burns in the angle of the eye.

Lasers are also being used in various stages of cataract surgery on a limited basis. Argon or krypton lasers are used in the treatment of retinal bleeding in diabetes, the wet type of macular degeneration, intraocular tumors or other types of retinal bleeding.

Lasers are used to remove skin lesions with the advantage of smaller incisions and less bleeding. The advantages of laser surgery are the ability to treat certain eye conditions that were not able to be adequately treated in the past, and the avoidance of surgical incisions into the eye, thus decreasing the complications of conventional surgical techniques and avoiding the inconvenience and expense of hospitalization. Laser use is performed in the outpatient setting and usually requires no anesthesia.

The excimer laser is used to treat refractive conditions—usually myopia (near-sightedness), astigmatism and some cases of hyperopia (far-sightedness) in a highly effective manner. For more precise cutting, carbon dioxide lasers are also used for oculoplastic and other plastic procedures, as well as general and urological surgery. This allows much surgery to be done with a minimum of bleeding, and dentists use infrared diode lasers in gum surgery. Lasers have had a major impact upon medicine by allowing treatment of many conditions in a quick, painless manner.

In the past, when the current prevalent method of phacoemulsification revolutionized cataract surgery, it was often erroneously referred to as laser removal of cataracts. However, lasers are evolving for use in cataract surgery and will probably become an essential part of this surgery in the future.

CHAPTER 54

You Wanna Cut What?

As physicians, we usually enjoy performing procedures and evaluations. However, the patient who's about to undergo these procedures and evaluations has certain expectations.

Physicians have the legal obligation to explain the indications, risks and alternatives of procedures. Don't be confused by the introduction of nurses and surgical schedulers or counselors into this equation. The use of these people and that expertise does not release physicians from the obligation to speak with you and to provide certain information. Every surgical procedure, or other procedures having risks, should have a notation, initialed by the physician, that the "indications, risks and alternatives" of the procedure have been discussed with the patient.

If you're accompanied by someone this should be marked in the chart. Then it should be mentioned that you understood what was said and would like to have (whatever) procedure performed, including, i.e., whether the work is to be done on the left or right side, and/or noting other geographic or descriptive details.

After a discussion with you, it should be noted if someone else—perhaps a nurse or surgical counselor—has also discussed the procedure., Even if noted or if recorded, a certain number of patients will say that the "doctor never spoke to me or discussed anything about the procedure with me." The physician should ask if you have any questions. The physician should never say: "This is minor and will be nothing significant from your viewpoint" as with even the most minor procedures, there can be a small percentage of problems.

You have a right to know what to expect and realistically what possible complications may occur.

You have an obligation to be interested to listen to the discussion and to ask questions as necessary. With operations on arms, legs, eyes, etc., that will be on one of two sites, you should be told that the operation will be on the "right arm" and that multiple people will ask as to what the operative site is and you should not be afraid to speak up.

If you're confused or don't understand, make sure that an individual with some rights of power of attorney is available and note this. You should also be told to call the office if other questions arise. In my career, I ended almost every office visit with "feel free to call me if you have any questions. If no one can answer them I will get back in touch with you."

CHAPTER 55

Seniors See Better Without Glasses—"Second Sight?"

The major situation in which this occurs is when a far-sighted individual develops cataracts. The change in the focusing lens of the eye makes the person temporarily less far-sighted or more near-sighted as the cataract develops.

In the early stages this acts to neutralize the far-sighted glasses, often enabling a person to dispense with the glasses for distant or near vision. As the cataract progresses, a point arrives where this "improved second sight" vision is lost.

Another condition in which the far-sighted

person may be able to read or see without glasses is the sudden onset of diabetes that might be otherwise unrecognized by the individual. This can come on extremely quickly and be quite alarming since everything in the distance is relatively suddenly blurred. It's easily diagnosed in the office and can be immediately reversed with new glasses. However, with control of the diabetes, the new glasses will no longer function well and the old glasses may not work as before.

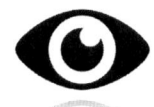

SECTION 3

Flat Out Staring

CHAPTER 56

Cataract Surgery— A Matter Of New Lenses

Almost all cataract surgery involves the implantation of an intraocular lens. This is an artificial lens implanted into the eye after removal of a cataract—and there are choices about what specific lens should be used. Cataract and implant surgery is amazingly successful for most individuals, often requiring no glasses (or minimal need for them) after surgery. The fact that glasses might be necessary usually is not a sign of poor results. It's usually a misunderstanding as to what to expect or a limitation of the implant used.

A single vision or astigmatism (toric) intraocular

lens will usually, but not always, require the use of glasses for near vision tasks unless a technique call monovision is used. In this situation one eye is corrected for near vision and one for distant vision. With monovision correction with single vision lenses you may still require some corrective glasses for driving or other distant tasks. For night driving and movies, many people prefer to wear glasses, which provide better binocularity and a slight improvement in distant vision.

You might want multifocal progressive lenses that you may wear as you like. These are especially helpful for computers and in between tasks. Requiring glasses after surgery is not a complication or a sign of poor surgery; rather it's the reality of dealing with cataracts.

If you have significant astigmatism, a toric lens may correct this astigmatism for distant vision and near vision. The same is true for the newer multifocal lenses, which correct both your near and distant vision, often allowing you to go without glasses completely. However, even with a multifocal lens you may have to wear glasses for some near or distant vision tasks. With some multifocal lenses there's increased glare and halo effect with driving; this may improve with time. These lenses, as well as multifocal lenses, are called premium lenses, and aren't paid for by Medicare

Performed on an outpatient basis, cataract surgery is normally a quick and efficient process, often taking under a half hour from start to finish. The surgeon must, of course, tell of you potential complications and risks. Those risks include:

- A rare infection.
- Possible glaucoma.
- Possible retinal detachment
- Possible corneal decompensation.

As with any procedure performed on older (or less commonly, younger individuals), stroke or death might ensue. Although it's extremely rare, there are situations in which this has occurred, and you must be told this.

Recognize also that there may be pre-existing conditions such as glaucoma, macular degeneration or corneal disease that may compromise the final results. In addition, pre-existing diseases of the eye or the body such as diabetes, glaucoma or macular degeneration may get worse and interfere with the final result.

CHAPTER 57

Macular Degeneration— Is There Hope?

Age-related macular degeneration (AMD) often doesn't have significant progression, and in turn causes minimal effect upon vision. However, what can be done to prevent it or to stop its progression when it occurs?

First, it's necessary to have an ophthalmologic exam at least every two years even if you don't have any eye complaints, since changes can be seen that may be precursors to macular degeneration, or macular degeneration can be diagnosed before it has affected the vision. For example, in people with 20/20 vision we often see little yellowish areas, called "drusen," in the area of the macula. A certain number of people with drusen will develop dry AMD—and we cannot predict which people or how long it might take.

In other individuals, we may see leaking blood vessels that grow under the macula and can cause a rapid loss of vision. They have a characteristic appearance and may be a form of the more serious wet AMD. In order to evaluate the status in more detail, it may be indicated to perform a fluorescein, or other dye study, to determine the status of the blood vessels at the back of the eye to determine if any treatment might be available.

This involves injecting a dye in a vein in the arm (in the office). The dye is then seen in the eye's blood vessels. Photographs are taken to analyze the type of degeneration and to determine and follow treatment. If no specific treatment is necessary, the patient is usually given an Amsler grid—a card with small squares which is used periodically. The patient looks at the card with one eye at a time and calls the ophthalmologist immediately if changes of vision occur, such as seeing a distortion of the squares or blocking out of some the squares. This is also used to monitor the vision after treatment.

What can be done now?

For the wet type of AMD, much progress has been made and, in some cases, the bleeding may be slowed down or stopped. The main treatment is called photodynamic therapy (PDT). A photosensitive substance is injected in a vein and concentrates in the area of the macula, following which it's activated by a special laser which causes clots to form and stop the leakage. If successful, it usually requires repetition every three months for one to two years. But be aware that this usually does not improve vision completely; rather it slows down the damage about 50 percent more than for those who have no treatment. More exciting is that this has stimulated research into a number of photosensitizing substances, which may be more effective and may be able to be used in other conditions.

For dry AMD the Age-Related Eye Disease Study (AREDS) has demonstrated that, in a number of patients who are at risk of developing dry AMD, may have their risk of developing the advanced disease reduced by about 25 percent and visual loss decreased by about 19 percent by the use of dietary supplements. These supplements contain antioxidants, vitamin C (500mg), vitamin E (400IU), beta-carotene (15 mg), zinc (80 mg) and copper (1.5mg). These are in a higher concentration than that found in most multivitamins. If you're a candidate for this, ask your ophthalmologist or optometrist for a specific recommendation since the same supplements used in the AREDS study are available commercially.

As with any substance, there may be side effects. Zinc may be responsible for urinary tract problems. Yellowing of the skin may result from the beta-carotene. Smokers may have a higher risk of lung cancer after using antioxidants. Discuss the advisability of using these oral supplements with your ophthalmologist and your primary care physician. In addition to the risks of cancer, smoking may be harmful to the macula—another reason to stop if you haven't yet done so. Carry out a healthy lifestyle with a good exercise program. Eat a well-balanced diet with green, leafy vegetables.

Again, it's important to recognize that the current treatments for dry or wet AMD aren't curative. The dietary supplements may slow down the progression for dry AMD and the photodynamic therapy may stop the bleeding and keep visual loss from progressing. While all vision is seldom lost—and despite the attempts to slow the process—there are situations in which some aspects of vision are lost. Often, most activities may be carried out outside of those that require sharp central vision such as driving or reading.

Total loss of vision almost never occurs, and there are many ways to maximize the remaining vision. Early on, large-print books, magazines and e-books will allow most people access to reading material. Later on, books on tape or CD are available free, allowing patients to keep up on many of the latest works of fiction and non-fiction. Large-print playing cards, watches, clocks, computers, etc., make life more comfortable. There are also magnifiers, either held in the hand or used on TV- type screens, which may allow use of standard print materials. A low-vision evaluation will determine the extent of your vision and what might be done to improve the vision.

Research is underway regarding the implantation of telescopic intraocular lenses, which may provide about 3X magnification. Currently such lenses create some loss of peripheral vision and take significant effort and time to learn to use them. Even though a patient has significant loss of vision as a result of macular degeneration, it's important to have periodic ophthalmologic or optometric exams in order to detect other conditions that may occur, such as cataract or glaucoma, Also, with the rapid advances in ophthalmology, you want to learn of anything that might help you as soon as possible.

This is an area which is constantly seeing new progress. Keep in touch with your eye care provider who can inform you when advances occur.

CHAPTER 58

What's "Lazy Eye" And How Is It Treated?

The brain can and will ignore double vision by causing one eye to be "suppressed" and not perform. This in turn can lead to "lazy eye" or amblyopia, a condition in which the eye is healthy but the vision is poor. If the two eyes aren't straight such as an eye turning in (is crossed), the vision in one eye may be suppressed in order to avoid double vision. This also may occur if only one eye is very near-sighted or very far-sighted. However, in about 50 percent of patients the eyes are straight.

In an infant, lazy eye may be suspected it the

child objects to having one eye covered, but not the other eye. This amblyopia causes no pain or difficulty and is usually detected during a routine eye examination or in school. I have seen patients in their forties and fifties who never knew that amblyopia was present until something happened, which caused them to have the vision in the good eye interrupted, at which time they noticed that the vision was poor in the other eye.

This is treated by correcting any need for glasses and by forcing the patient to use the amblyopic eye. This is usually accomplished by patching the good eye or blurring it with eye drops. The diagnosis and treatment should be started as early as possible, usually before about age five. The length of time for improvement may be days in an infant, or months or years in an older child. Occasionally it does not improve.

Surgical straightening is often performed, but this is primarily for cosmetic purposes and to attempt a restoration of binocular vision, not to treat the amblyopia. Although it's much more difficult to treat amblyopia over the age of ten to twelve years, improvement occasionally may occur later in life.

CHAPTER 59

A Vitreous What?

The eye contains fluids, with a major portion of the fluid being a thick jelly-like substance in the part of the eye behind the lens. This relatively clear substance is attached to the back of the eye in several places—and it's not unusual for it to pull free of its attachments, especially after the age of fifty years. This is called a "vitreous detachment."

When this suddenly happens some light flashes with possibly one or several floaters (or what appears to be a "fog" in front of one's vision) are noticed. However, the vision is relatively normal with no loss of side vision or significant blurring of vision. When this occurs, an examination by an ophthalmologist is necessary to determine the cause of the floater and light flashes, and also to make sure that no retinal tears or retinal detachment are present. Either present similar symptoms as the vitreous detachment, but both require immediate evaluation whereas the vitreous detachment exam is usually done on the same day or the next day with a follow-up exam in several weeks, and is then followed up by annual exams.

If a vitreous detachment is present there's no specific treatment. The patient is followed more closely in order to make sure that a retinal tear or detachment does not follow. Lasers have been used by some ophthalmologists to treat vitreous detachments, but this treatment is not generally accepted. Although the floaters and light flashes may disappear, what happens more commonly is that each remains and then ignored with the passage of time.

CHAPTER 60

What's That Floating In My Eye?

All of a sudden you notice a spot floating in your vision with some flashing lights. Is it serious? This is one of the more common questions that ophthalmologists hear. Usually the answer is simple—but you must get it checked out by your eye physician to make sure that it is or isn't serious. Fortunately, it usually isn't.

Several questions must be answered:

- Is this new?
- Is it just one floater or are there hundreds of little spots?

- Is this the first time you noticed it?
- Does it interfere with your vision?
- Do you have diabetes?

And what's a floater anyway?

The inside of the eye is filled with a gel-like substance called the vitreous. Although it's usually clear, a change in its consistency or bleeding may be noticed as a spot, spots or floaters. When there's some pulling on the retina, you may also notice flashing lights. The primary concern is that the floaters may be the first signs of a retinal detachment or bleeding in the eye.

Vitreous floaters were also discussed in the previous chapter.

On the other hand, it may be the sign of something more serious. The only way to be sure is to have your eyes examined. Usually the onset of new floaters, especially if they interfere with vision, is considered an emergency meaning that the patient is seen as soon as possible (this may vary after asking a few questions). But if there's interference with vision, the concern rises.

The more serious potential problems are retinal detachments and bleeding into the eye. With a retinal detachment, there's often a loss of some side vision, i.e., when covering the good eye, you may not see things off to the side of the affected eye and this loss may be accompanied by hundreds of little spots.

A retinal detachment means that the inside (seeing) layer of the eye (the retina) pulls off, causing the floaters (bleeding) in the eye. This is an emergency that must be seen immediately by the ophthalmologist. When seen in the office, drops are used to dilate the pupil (make it large), allowing us to look in the eye to diagnose the problem and decide upon the indicated treatment. If there's a lot of blood and the vision is poor, we may recommend bed rest to allow the blood to settle to allow an adequate view of the back of the eye.

Using an ultrasound machine will enable us to visualize what's happening behind the blood to determine if emergency surgery is necessary to remove the blood and reattach the retina. The longer that the retina is detached, the less likely vision may be restored.

If we can get a good view of the inside of the eye and are convinced that there's no retinal detachment, this is usually due to the common vitreous detachment. In this situation, there usually is only one floater and we may recommend avoiding vigorous activities for a short time, telling you to call immediately if there's an onset of many floaters. It's also recommended that you be re-evaluated in about a month to be sure that's nothing more serious. After that you can resume normal activities and have annual eye exams.

The floater is now a part of you. Although it's always there, you may learn to ignore it and notice it periodically such as when you look at the blue sky, etc. It may be evident as a "squiggly" line in your vision. It may appear as a "bug" which you want to brush away, but it remains—you look up, it moves down, you look to the left and it moves to the right, etc. Fortunately we usually learn to ignore it.

We get more concerned with patients that may have diabetes or bleeding problems since the presence of many floaters might be a sign of bleeding in the eye. This must be evaluated and the primary physician who cares for the diabetes should be notified to see if further medical evaluation must be done.

Currently, there's no accepted way of removing the floater if it's causing no problems. Going into the eye to remove the vitreous gel floater when there's no bleeding, retinal detachment or retinal problems usually will make the problem worse and isn't a good idea. Near-sighted individuals—or those people who have had cataract or other surgery of the inside of the eye—are more prone to floaters. In the absence of any disease, we usually get used to floaters and learn to ignore them. They are seen intermittently and cause no interference in vision.

There are other causes of flashing lights, most notably migraine headaches, which, if confined to the eye with flashing lights and with no disturbance of vision, require no treatment. If a headache occurs, this may be treated with medications. If there are questions, an exam is indicated to rule out any potentially blinding conditions.

CHAPTER 61

Why Do My Eyes Water A Lot?

To some degree eye watering depends upon your age and whether there's any disease present—but basically the tears do not drain through the tear ducts correctly, or the eyes produce too many tears. In young children the tear ducts may be blocked at birth. Most of these children respond to simple massage of the lids. If this doesn't solve the problem in several months, the tear ducts are opened with massage of the lids to express tears, with surgical opening being required relatively rarely. As we get older, the eyelids do not function as efficiently as they once did.

In this situation and in the situation where the tear ducts that carry the tears away from the eye may be blocked, there will be excess watering of the eyes.

Blocked tear ducts in infants may become infected and may require antibiotic medications or may require surgery to create an opening to carry the tears away into the nose. Since general anesthesia is typically used to open the ducts manual opening is tried first. In adults the tear ducts may also be abnormal and may require probing (opening) of the ducts at the eye doctor's office.

If the eyes don't produce sufficient tears or produce poor quality tears, small plugs may be easily placed in the tear ducts (in the office) to allow the tears to remain on the surface of the eye for longer periods of time.

Eyelids may become loose and turn in or out, either of which might cause tearing. Surgery of the lids is usually very successful.

With arthritis and other conditions in which the tears produced are either abnormal or are decreased in amount, it may be necessary to use one of a number of artificial tear substitutes. Occasionally special drops may be required to decrease irritation with its subsequent increased tearing, and it's rare that glasses will have any effect upon tearing. There are many diseases that may cause increased tearing: Conjunctivitis (pinkeye), glaucoma, eyelid abnormalities and many infections or other conditions may be responsible. When tearing becomes a problem, it should be evaluated in detail to determine if treatment is possible—and then determine which treatment.

CHAPTER 62

Will Ultraviolet Light Harm The Eyes?

Ultraviolet light (on the blue end of the spectrum) is most concentrated in sunlight. For many years it was believed that ultraviolet was filtered out by most glass and that it did not penetrate through the cornea and lens of the eye. However ultraviolet rays may penetrate into the eye and have a negative effect upon the lens and macula at the back of the eye, probably playing a role in the causation of cataracts or increasing their progression. Especially after cataract extraction—and with or without intraocular lens implantation—the retina may be more sensitive to ultraviolet light, whereby blood vessels may leak fluid with resulting blurred vision.

Because of this most implants now incorporate UV blocking. The most common injuries from ultraviolet light are the irritation to the cornea, with accompanying severe pain and redness, such as occurs in "snow blindness" or in tanning salons.

Many spectacle glasses and contact lenses, as well as most if not all intraocular lenses, also incorporate UV blocking. Sunglasses may vary and you must ask if there's ultraviolet protection. Simply being colored does not assure ultraviolet protection. Recognize that a certain amount of ultraviolet radiation passes through automobile windshields. In sensitive individuals it may be necessary to wear sunglasses when driving.

In occupations where one is exposed to harmful radiation, corneal burns, or damage to the retina, may occur. Adequate eye protection should be worn.

CHAPTER 63

Strokes Can And Do Affect The Eyes

The eyes may reveal that a person has a stroke or may tell the type of stroke and location of damage in the brain. This may be discovered on a routine eye exam before the individual notices any problems.

A condition known as "amaurosis fugax" may be the first sign of a stroke. This is a fleeting loss of vision in one eye whereby a person cannot see out of the eye for several minutes; then the vision returns to normal. In a similar way, there may be a short paralysis of one arm or side of the body.

On a routine eye exam, minute plaques of cholesterol in the vessels may indicate vessel damage and a minor or major stroke. The sudden onset of double vision or loss of part of the field of vision may be the only signs of a stroke or may be part of a major stroke involving several parts of the body.

When any of the above occurs, an ophthalmological or neuro-ophthalmological exam may give more detail about the stroke's exact location in the brain. Tests of side (peripheral vision) often will also reveal what part of the brain is involved in a stroke.

Following the peripheral vision, as well as the eye muscle movements, may be important in making a diagnosis as well as following the progress and hopeful improvement of a stroke. Loss of peripheral vision or double vision may require one to stop driving. This should be monitored by periodic exams since it may get better and enable resumption of driving.

CHAPTER 64

Thyroid Disease And Your Eyes

The best-known problem thyroid disease may create is bulging of the eyes, or exophthalmos due to infiltrates in the tissues behind the eye. This bulging may be more marked because of retraction of the eyelids, which also may be bulging and swollen. This should be measured and monitored closely to see if surgical decompression of the orbits should be carried out in order to avoid damage to the eyes

With involvement of the eye muscles, the eyes may not move well together, causing double vision, especially when looking upwards. Special glasses with prisms, or patching one eye may be needed. If stable for a long period of time, surgery might also be indicated. With extreme bulging the cornea (clear front window of the eye) may become dry, causing blurred vision. In these cases surgery may be required.

One of the confusing aspects of thyroid dysfunction is that the eye involvement may show up or progress in spite of good thyroid control and otherwise normal findings. It's essential that the primary care physician or endocrinologist cooperate with the ophthalmologist to coordinate management of the patient with thyroid abnormalities.

CHAPTER 65

Hey—You Have One Pupil Larger!

A certain number of people normally have one pupil larger than the other. It should be evaluated at some time in order to rule out any diseases. Trauma, i.e., a fall, or getting hit in the eye, are two of the most common reasons for a dilated (larger) pupil. Look at some old pictures to see if this is new or if it was present in the past. If there's an injury or a blow to the eye, the onset of a dilated pupil indicates that you should see an ophthalmologist to determine if there's any additional damage such as bleeding in the eye, a retinal detachment, or a cataract.

Other causes of a pupil becoming enlarged are strokes, diabetes, high blood pressure and brain tumors. These other causes usually are noticed by the individual and are often accompanied by double vision or decreased vision.

Horner's syndrome shows up as a small pupil associated with decreased sweating and a drooping eyelid on one side of the face. Neurological evaluations are carried out to try to find a cause for this.

Another common cause is the use of eye drops that were prescribed for someone else. These drops are usually in bottles with red tops. It's not a good idea to use anyone else's' drops or eye medications. The medication usually wears off in a matter of hours or days—but occasionally lasts up to two weeks. Depending upon the type of drops there may be more or less blurring of vision—usually for near vision.

A rare, but interesting cause of blurring is the exposure to certain perfumes when accidentally sprayed into the eye. For people who travel and want to take something to avoid motion or seasickness, use of scopolamine patches on the skin may result in one pupil being dilated with blurred vision for four to seven days.

Sudden or acute glaucoma may also cause the pupil to be dilated. This is usually associated with blurred vision, a red eye, and severe pain and requires immediate care by an ophthalmologist. Any change in pupil size requires a medical evaluation by an ophthalmologist in order to determine the cause and possible treatment.

CHAPTER 66

Retinitis Pigmentosa— Smaller And Smaller And Smaller

Retinitis pigmentosa refers to a group of conditions in which the retina at the back of the eye degenerates, causing decreased vision, especially at night. For some unknown reason, the rods and cones of the retina die. In the early stages the patient notices decreased night vision—and more than what normally occurs with aging. This is followed by reduced side or peripheral vision later.

This can start early in life and usually progresses gradually, enabling the individual to adjust. Some vision usually remains, even in the late stages. It usually runs in families and is inherited in one of a number of ways. Although it usually can be diagnosed during a regular eye evaluation, it might be necessary to do special testing to differentiate it from other causes of decreased vision.

There are many other types of retinal degenerations and night blindness that may occur. At the present time there's no known treatment for retinitis pigmentosa, and there's no vitamin treatment or medication that has had a beneficial effect.

There also has not been an eye transplant performed for this, or any other condition. Transplants of the clear cornea at the front of the eye may be performed, but this structure is not affected in retinitis pigmentosa. Although there's no evidence that light is harmful to the eyes, it's recommended to avoid long exposure to bright lights until more information is gathered. There's no evidence that use of the eyes will make things worse.

Low-vision aids such as special magnifying glasses or telescopes, large-print typewriters or computers, the wide angle mobility light, talking computers, and reading machines may assist individuals to maximize the use of remaining vision. Over a period of time the field of vision constricts and limits the visual field being seen to a very small area of vision—like looking through a minute hole where vision in a small area is visible, but no side or peripheral vision.

Injection treatments, which are offered in Russia and Cuba, aren't considered of any benefit by United States experts who are exploring gene therapy, stem cell treatments and other modalities. Efforts have been made to design glasses that can expand the side vision—but with limited success. A retinal prosthesis, or artificial retina, has been developed and should be improved with time. Although it does not allow the patient to actually see, it will allow the individual to discern some objects and to see contrasting objects in black and white. This has allowed some improved ambulation. The device is the Argus II and is made by Second Sight Medical Products as of February 2013.

For more information, contact: RP Foundation Fighting Blindness, 8331 Mindale Circle, Baltimore, Maryland 21207. The toll-free telephone number is 1-800-638-5682. This group has the latest information and is responsible for much research into the cause and possible treatment. The National Institutes of Health (NIH) also has information about the latest research at: *www.nih.gov.*

CHAPTER 67

I'm Not Sleepy— I Just Have Ptosis

Ptosis means that an eyelid is drooping. This might be present at birth or can come on any time during a person's lifetime. First, the individual must be evaluated to determine if there's a medical or a neurological cause that might require therapy. It might be the first sign of certain medical conditions (i.e., ptosis is relatively common in adult patients with diabetes and high blood pressure). Ptosis may come on rapidly in Bell's palsy or as the first sign of a stroke, brain tumor or other illness.

Ptosis is often present at birth with children.

If it's not severe and does not interfere with seeing, it might not be necessary to do anything. If it's cosmetically unacceptable, or if the child has to hold the head back to see, or if amblyopia "lazy eye" is present, then corrective surgery may be indicated early in life. The muscles that lift the eyelid respond quite well to corrective surgery. In adults the drooping lid may actually be low enough to interfere with vision. Ptosis may be due to aging changes or may also occur after eye surgery such as cataract surgery. But after medical causes have been eliminated, surgical treatment may be quite successful and results in some of our happiest patients.

CHAPTER 68

Eye Drops and You

Eye drops are medications that have specific actions and last for a variable period of time. However, drops may also be absorbed rapidly into the body and cause side-effects elsewhere. Some drops might be used once every week or two, whereas others might be necessary hourly or more often.

When using drops, usually only one drop is necessary since the second drop will overflow and wash out of the eye. Do not touch the dropper to the lashes (hold it away) since this would enable germs to enter the medication.

Absorption of some medications may cause elevation of blood pressure, difficulty breathing, slowing of the heart rate, nausea, etc. Patients may also have allergic reactions such as redness, itching, difficulty or cessation of breathing, etc. To decrease drop absorption, exert pressure, with the fingers, over the tear ducts at the inner corner of the eyelid for several minutes after instilling the drops.

Drops have effective actions that vary in time of onset and duration. For example, some drops will exert an effect for several minutes, while others may last hours to several weeks. Therefore, use drops at the intervals prescribed by your physician. Since drops are usually used for a specific purpose in an individual, it's important not to use them for other conditions or to use someone else's drops. If you have any untoward reaction or questions, discuss it with your physician or pharmacist immediately.

Drops are often very expensive. If generic drops are available, they may be significantly less expensive. In practice, we find that some generics (very few) are not as effective as the brand name. Ask you're your ophthalmologist or prescriber about this. He or she will usually know which ones not to use.

CHAPTER 69

How Does The Herpes Virus Affect The Eye?

Herpes infections of the eye are relatively common. Herpes simplex causes redness, tearing, irritation, blurring and severe sensitivity to light. Scarring of the cornea (the clear front part of the eye) may occur from herpes I infection, resulting in much loss of vision from damage to the cornea or the deeper parts of the eye. In severe cases a corneal transplant may be necessary in the future.

However, we have very effective eye drops to treat herpes simplex of the eye, recognizing that some cases will not respond to medication.

Genitourinary herpes infections are caused by the herpes II virus in 80 percent of cases and the herpes I virus in 20 percent. Although it rarely happens, the herpes I genito oral herpes is caused by herpes I in 80 percent of cases and may involve the eye. Herpes infections will cause the eye to be red, painful and sensitive to light with blurred vision. It's a serious condition that requires prompt evaluation and care by the ophthalmologist. In contrast, the less serious conjunctivitis, or "pinkeye" usually does not cause much pain, light sensitivity or blurring.

Ophthalmologists and patients have been fortunate to now have the first successful medications to successfully treat the herpes viral infections. In most cases, antiviral drops or ointments will cure the condition completely.

However, roughly 20 percent will have intermittent recurrences, requiring reinstitution of treatment with one of the several medications. If scarring of the cornea causes marked blurring of vision, a corneal transplant operation might be required to restore vision. Fortunately, the vast majority of ocular herpes infections respond favorably to medical treatment.

Herpes zoster (shingles) may also affect the

eye. It may cause painless redness as well as inflammation, which may affect the deeper structures of the eye causing damage to vision. If you have herpes zoster and develop eye redness you should be evaluated quickly to see if the eye is actually involved.

CHAPTER 70

Can Juvenile Arthritis Affect The Eyes?

Juvenile rheumatoid arthritis occasionally is associated with uveitis of the eye. Uveitis is an inflammation of the eye whereby cells leak out of blood vessels. Similar inflammation in an adult usually is associated with marked redness of the eye, pain, sensitivity to light and blurred vision. Unfortunately these warning signals may be absent in children who may only experience little or no discomfort.

Diagnosis of this uveitis requires the specialized equipment of the ophthalmologist. Fortunately it does not occur often. When it does, treatment is the use of cortisone eye drops, dilating drops and possibly oral steroids to reduce the inflammation and relax the pupil. Close observation is necessary to prevent the potential complications of glaucoma and cataract.

Children with juvenile rheumatoid arthritis should have regular ophthalmological exams to diagnose eye involvement as early as possible in order to treat it early and avoid major eye complications—which can include loss of vision.

Adult arthritis usually affects the eyes by causing general irritation and dryness of the eyes.

CHAPTER 71

What's "Pressure" In The Eye?

T he eye is similar to a ball or a balloon that contains fluid. Since the eyeball must be fairly firm in order to keep its relatively round shape, the amount of hardness or softness (pressure) may be measured by any one of several instruments placed on the eye or via a puff of air blown at the eye. These instruments are called tonometers. This testing of pressure is often called the "glaucoma test" since elevated pressures in the eye may cause the damage to the optic nerve with loss of side vision and known as glaucoma.

All eyes contain fluid—and this means that all eyes normally have "pressure." Concern is raised when the pressure is high enough to the extent that ocular damage might occur. Since we're all individuals, the eye pressure in different persons will vary. In addition the pressure varies in the same individual during a twenty-four-hour period—called diurnal variation. It's occasionally necessary to measure the pressure during the night in situations where the pressure rises to abnormal levels, resulting in damage to the eye.

What's safe for one individual might not be safe for another. It's in the province of the ophthalmologist or optometrist to evaluate the pressure test with other tests to determine whether treatment is necessary. The pressure test is only a small, but very important, part of detecting glaucoma. It can often be the first step in finding individuals at an early stage when it may be possible to institute treatment and prevent the damage and visual loss that might occur from glaucoma. It's not a substitute for a complete eye examination since glaucoma might be present in spite of a normal "pressure test" due to the normal variations of pressure. There is also a low-tension glaucoma that would be missed if only the pressure is measured.

Most blindness from glaucoma would be preventable if the disease was detected early enough, thereby emphasizing the importance of regular eye exams, especially over the age of thirty-five years when pressure elevations and glaucoma become more common.

CHAPTER 72

Can AIDS Affect The Eye?

The eye has been involved in about 75 percent of AIDS patients in the past. This is less likely today since the newer AIDS treatments are available. At the back of the eye (the retina), hemorrhages and white spots because of circulation problems may occur. Actual infection of the retina by the cytomegalovirus, as well as other infections, can occur and lead to severe damage to the retina and loss of vision. Medications have limited success in treating these infections. This is rarer with the newer treatments.

Kaposi's sarcoma, a cancer that may occur

in association with AIDS, can also involve the eyelids or conjunctival covering of the eye. Lastly, if AIDS affects the brain, it may interfere with vision by damaging the areas of the brain that deal with vision. It's important to detect the eye problems as early as possible in order to initiate treatment for a treatable complication of being infected by the AIDS virus.

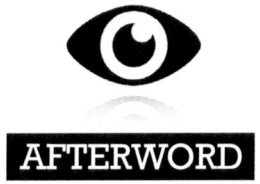

AFTERWORD

The goal of this book has been to make you a better patient by understanding how to deal with the medical system and how to care for your eyes. It is also meant to help you understand some of the conditions that might affect your vision. To learn more or contact the author, visit *www.DrFrankWeinstock.com*.

ABOUT THE AUTHOR

Dr. Frank Weinstock, M.D., F.A.C.S., is a board certified ophthalmologist, Fellow of the American College of Surgeons, and the author of eight other books, including *Contact Lenses Fitting: A Clinical Text Atlas*, which has been translated into German and Spanish. He is also the author of hundreds of articles on related eye and health topics. Dr. Weinstock is a professor at Northeast Ohio Medical University, an affiliate clinical professor in the Charles E. Schmidt College of Biomedical Science at Florida Atlantic University, and a volunteer professor of ophthalmology at the University of Miami Leonard M. Miller School of Medicine. He has received multiple honors, including the Lifetime Achievement Award and Senior Honor Award of the American Academy of Ophthalmology as well as the Senior Honor Award of the Contact Lens Association of Ophthalmologists. He also has done notable volunteer work in El Salvador, Nepal and Papua, New Guinea.

Other Works
By Frank J. Weinstock, M.D., F.A.C.S.

Clinical Eye Care Forms

Contact Lens Dispensing

Contact Lenses Fitting: A Clinical Atlas

The Dermatology Office Manual

The Family Practice Office Manual

Geriatric Opthalmology

HIPPA and Compliance

Management and Care of the Cataract Patient

The Ophthalmologist's Office: Planning and Practice

The Opthalmology Office Manual

The Urology Office Manual

Your Medical Future: Make the Right Decision Now

www.DrFrankWeinstock.com